Where Your Mind Goes Energy Flows

A Self-Healing Manual for the Mind and Body

by Michèle Bourgeois B.Sc.N., M.Ed.
illustrated by Valerie Woelk

World rights reserved. This book or any portion thereof may not be copied or reproduced in any form or manner whatever, except as provided by law, without the written permission of the author, except by a reviewer who may quote brief passages in a review.

The author of this book does not dispense medical advice or prescribe treatment. The author's approach is holistic, focusing on the reader as a complex, dynamic and unique being of body, mind and spirit. This information is complementary to any medical treatment that the reader undertakes. The author does not assume responsibility for how the reader chooses to use this information. The advice of your physician is strongly recommended.

Copyright 2017 Michèle Bourgeois B.Sc.N., M.Ed.

Edited by Karina Sinclair

1st edition 2018

ISBN-13: 978-1-7751844-0-9 (Paperback)

ISBN-13: 978-1-7751844-1-6 (ePub)

ISBN-13: 978-1-7751844-2-3 (Mobi)

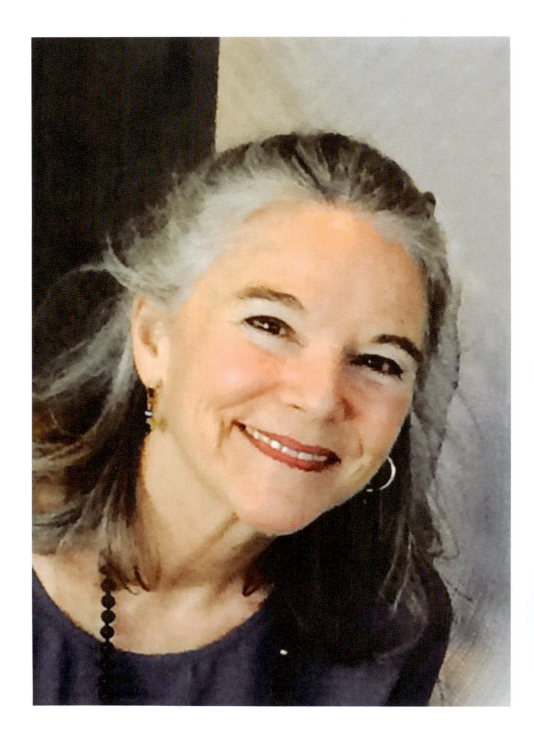

About the Author

Michèle Bourgeois B.Sc.N., M.Ed. is an energy healing practitioner with over 40 years of combined experience in the traditional medical field and alternative and complementary holistic therapies. Her skills range from bedside nursing and teaching, to health promotion and education, to program planning and implementation and professional energy healing. She has a Bacaleaureate in the Science of Nursing and a Masters in Education.

She has pursued the study of energy healing science at the premier institute of hands-on energy healing and personal transformation, the Barbara Brennan School of Healing. She graduated from the program in 2002 and is a certified Brennan Healing Science Practitioner. She is also the co-founder of the Grace Touch Healing—Living from Grace Program in Canada.

Michèle's belief about healing is that each of us is his or her own healer; that healing comes primarily from within. Her approach is holistic, focusing on you as a complex, dynamic and unique being of body, mind and spirit.

She has had an active energy healing practice since 2002. As an energy healing practitioner, teacher, and holistic nurse, Michèle is well known for her warmth and kindness as well as her clarity, insights, and healing skills. **wwww.turningpointhealing.com**

About the Illustrator: Valerie Woelk

Valerie has been a commercial freelance illustrator since 1997 doing a wide assortment of work in automotive, motorcycle & building murals, book illustration, along with various commissions in oil, watercolour, acrylics and black & white. Her work is described as realistically surreal and colourful. This project was a joyful, creative, and cooperative effort allowing this style to blossom. Valerie also did all the book graphic design typesetting and layout. **www.valeriewoelk.com**

Acknowledgements

*I want to thank my clients and students of the past 20 years. I have continually been inspired by their courage and tenacity. Without all I have learned working with them, this body of work would not have been developed. I am deeply grateful to each and every one of them for their trust and confidence over the years.
You know who you are!*

I want to thank Donna Evans-Strauss, my friend, teacher, mentor, colleague and co-founder of the Living from Grace Program in Canada. Without this program and Donna's positivity, enthusiasm and encouragement this book would not have had the platform to manifest.

I want to thank Susan Beach, my friend, for her positive outlook about writing, words of wisdom, and encouragement to work on this book from its inception. She is also is the editor of the Self-healing Meditation Card Set that accompanies this book project.

I want to thank Valerie Woelk, my friend and very talented artist. With my input about the human energy field and the anatomy of the body, she was able to transform my ideas into the beautiful images of the body systems in this book project. Her many skills, encouragement and tenacity have been a major support to me through the publishing process.

I want to thank my husband, children and extended large family for their endless and unconditional support of my work and especially this book project.

Last but not least, I want to thank Dr. Barbara Ann Brennan, my teacher of energy healing science, and the Barbara Brennan School of Healing for the rigorous, supportive, cutting edge and professional program that it is. My time in the program truly was a turning point in my life.

Contents

Introduction -- **10**

Chapter 1

The Heart and Circulation System ---------------------- **16**
Connection, Communication and Love
Self-Healing Meditation for **the Heart**-------------------------------- **24**
Self-Healing Meditation for **the Circulation System**------------------ **25**

Chapter 2

The Nervous System -- **26**
Communication and Control
Self-Healing Meditation for **the Nervous System** ---------------------- **33**

Chapter 3

The Respiratory System -------------------------------------- **34**
Giving and Receiving Life
Self-Healing Meditation for **the Respiratory System** ------------------ **41**

Chapter 4

The Immune System -- **42**
Discernment and Protection
Self-Healing Meditation for **the Immune System** ---------------------- **49**

Chapter 5

The Digestive System -- **50**
Nourishment and Contentment
Self-Healing Meditation for **the Digestive System** -------------------- **57**

Chapter 6

The Endocrine System -------------------------------------- **58**
Balance and Coordination
Self-Healing Meditation for **the Endocrine System** ------------------- **67**

Chapter 7

The Musculoskeletal System --- 68
Support and Mobility
Self-Healing Meditation for the Musculoskeletal System --- 77

Chapter 8

The Skin System --- 78
Boundary of Reception and Protection
Self-Healing Meditation for the Skin System --- 85

Chapter 9

The Urinary System --- 86
Elimination and Balance
Self-Healing Meditation for the Urinary System --- 91

Chapter 10

The Reproductive System --- 92
Creativity and Sexuality
Self-Healing Meditation for the Reproductive System --- 101

Chapter 11

The Sensory System --- 102
Perceiving and Discerning
Self-Healing Meditation for the Sensory System --- 109

Chapter 12

The Whole Body --- 110
Self-Healing Meditation for the Whole Body --- 112
Conclusion --- 114
Appendix --- 118
Chakras
References --- 120
Self-Healing Meditation Cards 12-Piece Set --- 122

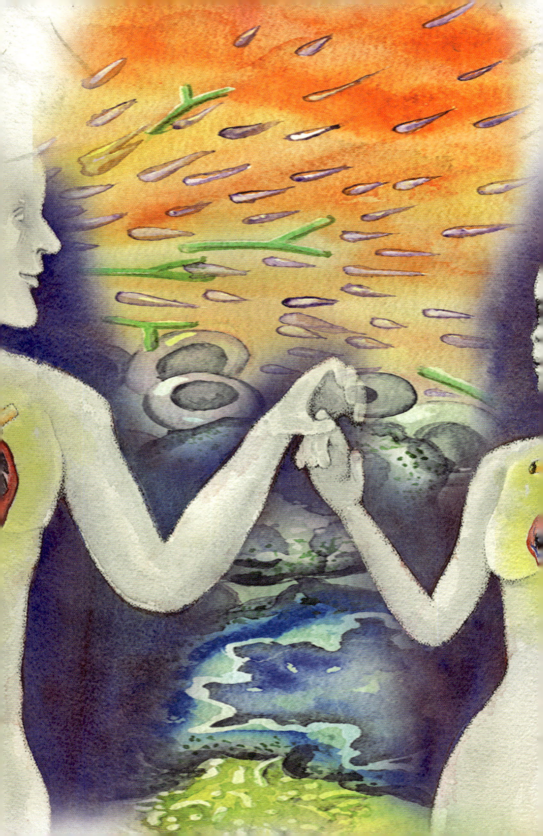

Introduction

When we understand the physical nature of our body systems and what they represent from a holistic perspective, we are more consciously connected to our overall health.

This manual provides you with a brief overview of the anatomy, physiology and the mind-body connection of human body systems. Twelve body systems have been identified. It is important to note that these body systems work together as a whole. Each system is dependent on the other systems, much like we human beings are interconnected with each other in our families, communities, countries and on earth.

Each chapter begins with a brief description of the anatomy and physiology of a human body system. Prevailing concepts from the current literature on psycho-emotional aspects of health and illness (referred to as the mind-body connection) are then discussed. The chapter concludes with a Self-Healing meditation focused on the respective body system. This is meant to be a hands on, easy to read, practical manual. To support and further your study of the psycho-emotional connections of health and illness, I encourage you to have a look at the references included at the end of this book. For further information about the anatomy and physiology of each body system, I direct you to any medical textbook or to the internet, where there are countless educational resources and audiovisual aids on the anatomy and workings of the body. Please note that the word "mind" in the context of this book refers to the part of a person that enables them to be consciously aware of the world and their life experiences; to think, to feel, and access their beliefs and emotional patterns.

The connection between our emotions and our health is not a new idea. Your family doctor may ask you what is happening in your personal and emotional life when you come in complaining of symptoms such as headaches or stomachaches. In the allopathic medical world, there is a strong focus on a scientific evidence-based approach to health care. Antibiotics and surgeries do save lives. Competent emergency health care certainly decreases morbidity and mortality rates. Genetics as well play a huge role in health and illness. However, in our diligence to look at health issues more objectively, we have underestimated the vital role of psycho-emotional aspects in health and illness. In the past few decades, the study of the relationship between mind and body has been slowly emerging. It is my hope that with this body of work, a more inclusive and balanced understanding of why we get sick, and how to heal ourselves can be restored.

A holistic view to health and how we care for the sick was perhaps better understood by our ancestors. As a child, I can remember that when I would tell my mother I had a stomachache, she would ask me what I was worried about while she laid her hand on my tummy. Even as an adult when I would talk to my mother about having a headache or a cold, she would ask me about my work or how busy was I at school.

There are countless everyday examples that illustrate how emotions and our psychological state affects the physiology of our body. One of the most obvious examples is how sadness and extreme happiness triggers the production of tears. I often wonder how actors can make themselves cry. I suspect they have to bring to mind something personal that makes them feel very sad. Other examples include how we flush easily when embarrassed or the way our heart races when we feel a surge of love for another person. I inevitably have skin problems during times of emotional stress in my life. Take a moment now to think back to how your body felt when you experienced your first kiss, watched a horror movie, wrote an exam for a difficult course, or before you have given a public speech. How does

Allow the mind-body connections to be simply suggestions for consideration. Avoid labelling disorders with psycho-emotional causes or casting blame on yourself or others for causing the illness.

your body react to something in your life that is very sad, threatening, loving, happy or stressful?

The mind-body connection is wired into the nervous system and the brain. Consider the fight or flight reaction of the nervous system, and its part in connecting emotional content and physical changes in the body. When frightened by a real or imagined danger, the physiological fight or flight response is switched on automatically. Consider the effect that meditation has on the brain and body, and how this can in turn affect mood changes. There are several research studies which suggest that there are physical benefits to be had from the calming effects of meditation.

In my years working as a nurse on various specialty units in the hospital, I often wondered why many patients with similar physical health problems, such as gastrointestinal or heart problems, would seem to display similar emotional issues or attitudes about life. You may have wondered how emotions affect your physical health. These considerations are only a part of the overall picture of health and illness but nonetheless play a role. I believe we are doing ourselves a disservice if we ignore the mind-body connections of health and illness.

As you read through the mind-body connections of each body system, allow them to be simply suggestions for consideration. Avoid labelling disorders with psycho-emotional causes or casting blame on yourself or others for causing the illness. We often tune out the emotional components of our physical problems. If we give ourselves time to listen carefully to the body and mind, we can access our intuition to help us see a more personal and holistic picture of the physical problem. There are often emotional growth opportunities through an illness. Underlying states of consciousness can surface at quiet times or during meditation that can help you through a health challenge.

From a scientific point of view, evidence is emerging about the power of the mind. The principles of the quantum field theory in physics supports the assertion that we can influence our physical health through our thoughts, beliefs and emotional patterns. At the quantum level, your body, which is made of energy, is constantly changing and is under the direction of your conscious awareness. (West, 2014).

This information and these meditations guide you to explore the connections between your personal issues, thoughts, emotions, and your physical health. The self-healing body system meditations at the end of each chapter can help you sink into a quiet place. You may get a glimpse of the deeper meaning underlying your physical health problem. This can help you use your innate healing abilities to restore your physical, mental and spiritual health.

Take your time as you examine the images and read about the body systems. Try the self-healing meditative exercises included. It is best to work with one system at a time. With practice, it will become easier to connect with your own body systems. Overtime, you may find that insights about your physical and emotional well-being emerge naturally. Disease patterns may begin to dissolve and new ways of dealing with your health or illness may become evident.

Introduction

"Your ability to create a focus of attention is not just a cerebral, or brain, activity. It is an activity on many levels of consciousness. Wherever you place your attention within your body, or within the energy field of your body, there is an immediate flow of subtle energy to that point, or area, which has an enlivening effect upon the cells of your body, and/or the luminous light fibres that comprise your **energy body***." (Kenyon, April 18, 2005.)*

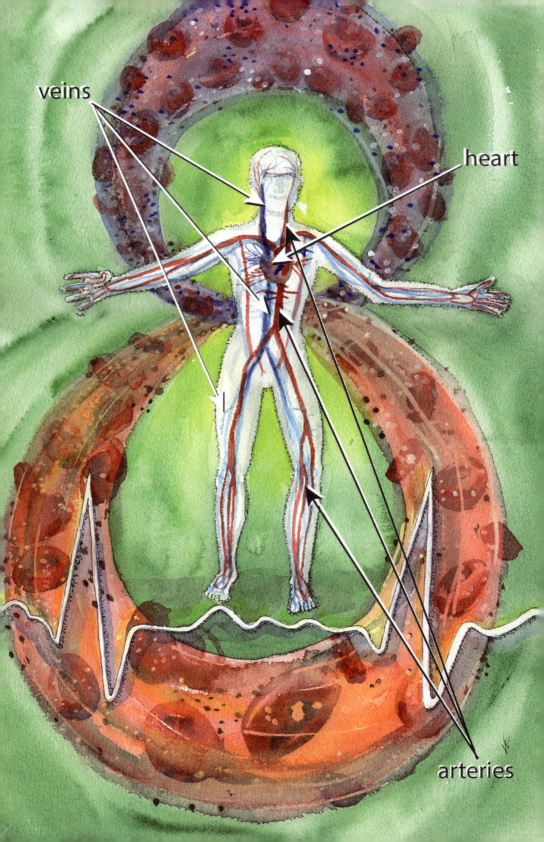

Chapter 1
The Heart and Circulation System
Connection, Communication and Love

The heart is referred to by many healers of ancient and more modern healing modalities as the master of the body, mind and spirit. When the heart is healthy, the rest of the body can come into whole health and balance.

Anatomy & Physiology of the Heart & Circulation System

The heart works closely with all the body systems but has a very close, functional connection to the respiratory system. The respiratory system provides the blood with oxygen; and the circulatory system, of which the heart is the core, transports the oxygen-rich blood to the cells. Humans can live for weeks without food, days without water, but only a few minutes without oxygen. The circulatory system transports oxygen from the lungs to the cells and then removes the waste products from cells. The bloodstream also circulates; cells that defend against infections, hormones produced by glands to regulate the body's workings, nutrients from food, chemicals, ions, gases, and heat throughout your body. It is a transportation and delivery system. If you are running, it moves oxygen down to your legs, and moves lactic acid (the chemical that gives your muscles that burning sensation when worked hard) out of your legs. It moves heat from your body core to your toes, fingers, and head on a cold day. It also distributes nutrients from your digestive system throughout your body, feeding your bones, nerves, organs, and other tissues in your body.

The heart and the blood vessels are the main structures of the heart and circulation system. There are arteries, veins and millions of microscopic blood vessels called capillaries, that distribute blood to the individual cells.

Blood pressure is the pressure of the blood flowing through the heart and circulatory system. The pressure fluctuates depending on how much blood we need pumped through at any given moment. If our blood pressure stays high even when we are relaxed, this is a problem because constant high blood pressure is hard on the heart and blood vessels, especially the tiny ones in the brain. Strokes are often caused by these tiny blood vessels in the brain bursting under constant high pressure. Your blood pressure normally remains fairly stable because the body adjusts the resistance of the arteries; either widening or narrowing them as needed, to prevent the blood pressure from swinging wildly.

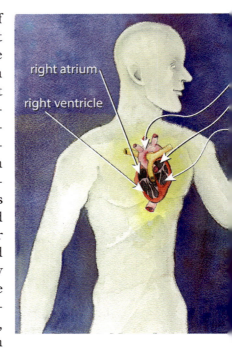

The Mind-Body Connection of the Cardiovascular System

The heart has a powerful electromagnetic field, and emanates more electricity and magnetism than any other organ in the body, including the brain.

The heart as master of the body, mind and spirit is home to our emotions and thus has a powerful connection to our psyche. For that reason, we really have to go beyond thinking of it in a mere physical sense. The heart receives information from the environment first, even before the brain does. (Wolf & Becker, 2009) The heart has its own nervous system that can sense, feel, remember and

The heart receives information from the environment first, even before the brain does.

process information independently from the brain. It is modulated by emotional patterns that become imprinted on its magnetic field. It is the generator of all emotions – your passion, fear, hurt, joy, gratitude, yearnings and anger. All these emotions are expressed from the heart throughout the mind and body. Because the heart is responsible for blood circulation, it is capable of sending emotional signals via the blood to all other body systems and right into the cells. (The HeartMath Institute, 2013; Wolf & Becker, 2009)

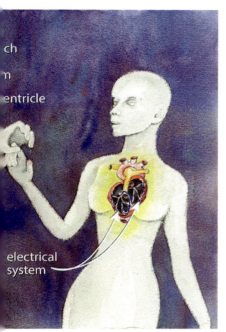

Why is it important to understand this? Because if the heart metabolizes emotion how can it not be physically affected by what we feel and how we act in our lives? In addition, does this mean that emotions that affect the heart, then get pumped through the body via the blood circulation?

The human heart, is an empathic centre and radiates and receives invisible frequencies of energy and consciousness. (Brennan, 2017) These energies can have a direct effect on your blood pressure, nervous system, lungs, organs, brain, and really your whole body. Thus, the heart becomes a major communication centre between the brain and all other systems of the body. Noted author Louise Hay (1998) even goes so far as to assert that heart problems suggest long-standing emotional issues such as lack of joy, or holding onto strain and stress. A heart attack, she says, is really about "squeezing all the joy out of the heart in favour of money or position (p.48)." Dr. Andrew Weil (1998), the au-

> *You have the natural ability to send healing energy messages from your heart to others.*

thor who champions integrative medicine, expresses a similar belief that the people most at risk of heart attack are those who cannot give and receive love in a nurturing way.

Consider a time when you were around someone who was anxious. How did their anxiety make your heart feel? Were there visible signs of anxiety or did you pick it up in a different way? Now consider a time when you were in the presence of someone who was filled with joy. How did the frequency of joy make your heart feel? These emotional expressions are all transmitted via the invisible field that exists between others and ourselves. (Brennan, 2017) Sometimes, you may even feel anxiety before an event actually happens just as a new mother may awake a few minutes prior to her newborn child crying to be fed or changed.

> *Fear is often referred to as the opposite of love.*

There is an intricate web of communication transmitting messages to and from your heart centre. You have the natural ability to send healing energy messages from your heart to others. The very frequencies of your heart can have a direct effect on how another person feels. This knowledge offers you the opportunity to build healthy and healing relationships. Our heart is the main communicator and receiver of emotions, and thus is the epicentre of relationship.

Barbara Brennan (1988), explains that the fourth chakra governs the heart and circulation system and is the energy centre through which we love. "When this centre is functioning, we love ourselves, our children, our mates, our families, our pets, our friends, our neighbours, our countrymen, our fellow human beings and all our fellow creatures on this earth." (p. 76)

It sends and receives empathic expressions; feelings of joy and happiness, sadness and grief or frustration and anger, just to name a few. It sends signals to our brain to activate different responses that vary greatly from peacefulness to heightened anxiety. Our hearts can even empathetically receive messages from our environment that are beneath our conscious awareness. (Brennan, 2017; Pearsall, 1998; Zukav, 2001; Wolf & Becker, 2009)

The heart is seen as a symbolic representation of love that seems to be universally accepted. The connection between the heart and love is deeply rooted in our collective psyche. When we experience conflict or abuse, hurt or loss, as we all inevitably will at some point; there is a potential for us to close down our hearts and emotionally lock others out, including ourselves. We may even feel we don't need love as we experience a lack of trust, or feel uncaring, prejudiced, shallow, hateful or fearful. Fear is often referred to as the opposite of love. When we feel fear our heart tends to close off. We would do well if we learned how to think with our hearts rather than with our heads. Pearsall, in his book The Heart's Code (1998), writes "...I have very little doubt that the heart is the major energy centre of my body and a conveyor of a code that represents my soul" (p.4).

Here are some questions to consider

...when working with your heart & circulation system.

Take a moment to consider what it would feel like to experience rejection, anger, or hatred, coming from a loved one.

Does it make your heart beat faster or slower?

How does the heart communicate to other parts of your body and your brain when it is under distress?

For some people negative emotions cause a shortness in breathing. For others it may cause heartburn, heart palpitations or even stomach or bowel problems.

Imagine love and acceptance coming from others toward you.

How do you feel?

Do you take it in?

Do you mistrust it?

Do you shut it off and judge the other?

Sometimes we reject the very thing we are craving.

What happens when you let go of mistrust and judgments?

Consider for a moment how love and acceptance flows toward you and out toward others.

How willing are you to open your heart and let love in and give love to others?

The Heart and Circulation System

If you're finding it hard to grasp the concept of the heart's emotional influence, think about this:

> *One of the most important medical achievements of our time is the heart transplant. While it was indeed an amazing scientific feat, this treatment really captured our imaginations as we learned that the recipient of the heart transplant often experiences the emotions of the donor. It was the first concrete proof that this vital organ did more for us than just pump blood. (Shapiro, 2006; Pearsall, 1998)*

Self-Healing Meditation for
the Heart
Love and Connection

Bring the image of the heart to your awareness. Place your right hand on your lower belly and your left hand on your chest. Connect with your heart and tell it you completely support all it has done for you, and that it is strong and capable of supporting you further in your life.

Feel and listen to the rhythm of your heart beat. Take a deep breath. Allow your heart to peacefully send and receive loving messages to every cell of your body and to all the people in your life. May you sit gently with your heart issues as you let new possibilities open up for you. There is waiting for you, more joy and true freedom! Relax and let it come to you.

Let your heart know that you have complete trust and confidence in its natural ability to bring health, love and connection to your life and your relationships. Let your heart beat the rhythm of your soul's longings and wisdom throughout your body, mind and spirit many times, each minute. Let your mind put into action, what it is that your heart wisdom beats out to you each moment.

May you know the blessings of your heart light's code.

Self-Healing Meditation for
the Circulation System
Connection and Communication

Bring the image of the heart and circulation system into your awareness and let it flow into your body. Place your right hand on your lower belly to connect to the circulatory system of the lower body, and your left hand on your chest to connect to your heart and the circulatory system of the upper body.

Imagine the main purpose of your heart is to regularly beat out blood that is saturated with unconditional love. This is the power of love happening in every moment!

Listen to your heart beat. Connect to the rhythm of your heartbeat and imagine your blood circulating with ease throughout your body. Allow your heart to peacefully transport and deliver life giving signals to every cell of your body. May you lie lightly with your issues so that they can be easily dissolved.

Let the loving energy in your heart upwell. Let your heart beat out the song of your soul as it connects to every part of your body through your blood, bringing a coherent rhythm of whole health and happiness throughout. Let your heart and circulation system know that you have complete trust and confidence in their natural abilities to bring health, communication and connection to your life.

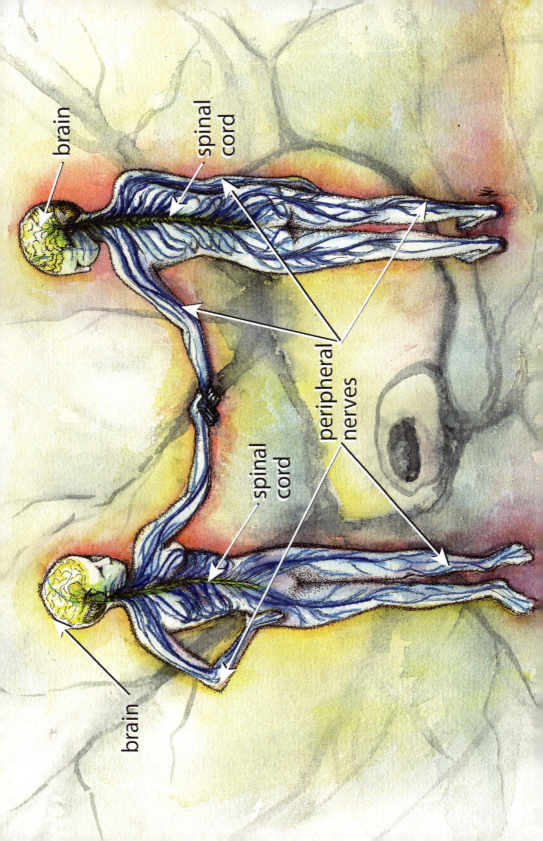

Chapter 2
The Nervous System
Communication and Control

The nervous system consists of a vast network of nerve cells that make up a phenomenal communication system in the human body. Information is constantly being sent and received through the brain, spinal cord and nerves within the body and between the body and the outside world. It can be likened to a super communication highway system and control centre. The nervous system is about communication and control.

The brain sends messages down the spinal cord, which branches out to nerves reaching all other systems of the body. These messages provide us with motor and sensory abilities, as well as other various physical functions. The brain provides us with mental functions as well, which is unique to human beings. Thought processes such as planning and problem solving, processing and storing emotions, and the creation of and storing memories are all happening here in the brain.

Anatomy and Physiology of the Nervous System

In the image of the nervous system you can see the brain in yellow, spinal cord in green and the nerves in blue. It is a beautiful network of nerve activity, rooted in the brain. With this overall image of the nervous system in mind, let us take a closer look at all the parts of the nervous system.

The Nerve Cell

The nerve cell, or neuron, is the basic structural unit of the nervous system. It consists of a cell body and extending fibres called dendrites and axons. The dendrites are the fibres that receive impulses from the axons of other nerve cells. Nerve cells possess the reciprocal characteristic properties of receptivity and conductivity. There are also chemical messengers involved in facilitating and inhibiting these communication processes. Nerve cells are highly qualified to communicate messages accurately.

The Brain

Brain tissue is made of a network of nerve cells. These nerve cells are coated with myelin, which is a white sheath that allows nerve impulses to travel more rapidly, facilitating communication. The brain is the central control system of the body. The largest region of the brain, the top part, is the cerebrum which is divided into left and right halves (cerebral hemispheres). The left side of the brain controls motor and sensory activity of the right side of the body, and the right side of the brain controls motor and sensory activity of the left side of the body. The left side of the brain is linear, rational and logical, and controls rapid thinking processes. The right side of the brain is visual, creative, sensitive, and relational. There are also centres in the brain that govern speech, sight, hearing, smell, and touch. The various centres in the brain work in concert with all other body systems such as the cardiovascular, endocrine and digestive systems. The brain also receives and responds to stimuli from the outside world to keep us healthy and performing to our potential. Deep within the inner brain, thought patterns and emotional habits get rooted. Distorted emotional patterns can affect our health and wellness negatively.

The brain stem is at the base of the brain and is made up of all the myelinated nerve fibres from the cerebrum and connects the upper parts of the brain to the spine. The cerebellum, at the back and base of the brain, is the centre of body coordination. It blends and coordinates voluntary muscle movements and helps one maintain an upright posture.

The Spinal Cord and Nerves

The spinal cord travels from the brain stem, through a long opening down the length of the back bones (spinal column). Spinal nerves emerge from the brain stem and through various openings from each side of the spinal column. Imagine the spinal cord as being one main communication track with spinal nerves branching out down the length of it. These nerves then divide into many smaller nerves, reaching out to all structures of the body, such as the bones, skin, muscles and organs. Messages, in the form of nerve impulses, are communicated to and from the body systems and the brain through the spinal nerves.

Some nerves control sensations and movements; and some nerves, called autonomic nerves, govern involuntary functions. These autonomic nerves control nerve impulses that regulate many involuntary physiological activities, such as the heartbeat, breathing and digestive functions. Some of these nerves, (the parasympathic nerves) regulate involuntary functions to maintain balance and functioning of the organs. The other autonomic nerves (the sympathetic nerves) take over during times of imbalance and stress. They govern the fight or flight (stress) responses during times of crisis. The stress response is triggered when one perceives a threat to life or safety, as well as when one experiences negative emotions such as fear, regardless whether the perceived fear is real or not. Imagined fears can trigger the stress response, and frequent or prolonged stress responses take their toll on the body over time. (Maté, 2004)

The Mind-Body Connection of the Nervous System

This vast superhighway communicates various messages of health or distress to every system and organ of the body. If our thoughts and emotions are unhealthy, soon our nervous system

The primary intention of the nervous system is to provide communication and control: to facilitate accurate and healthful communication of information throughout the body...

responds with anxiety and duress sending messages out, and creating chemicals to counterbalance the stress. It wants to bring the body into balance and right order. The nervous system is in close communication with the heart which is our emotional centre, as well as with the whole body. It signals us when something is wrong. For example, we might get a backache, a headache, or a stomachache as a warning sign to slow down and observe what is happening.

The primary intention of the nervous system is to provide communication and control: to facilitate accurate and healthful communication of information throughout the body, within the body itself, and between the outer world and self. All of the seven major chakras play a role in supplying the nervous system with vital energy especially the third chakra. (Brennan, 1993) When the nervous system is in good health, perceptions and nerve transmissions are accurate, smooth, direct, and timely. Nerves pick up messages from the physical body, as well as from our emotions and thoughts, and transmit them to the brain. The brain then responds and sends reactive messages to the body. (Shapiro, 2006)

> ...joy, happiness, loving kindness, and forgiveness increases the healthy flow of nervous functions...

Within this complex system numerous communications are going on. Blockages or faults in any one area can affect other areas or create a system failure. Blockages can include emotions such as fear, panic, mistrust, and shame, not to mention physical injuries or disruptions due to a disease. These blockages can all undermine the normal functioning of the nervous system. "In the same way, joy, happiness, loving kindness, and forgiveness can increase your well-being, leading to a balanced, calm, and healthy nervous system." (Shapiro, 2006, p. 154) If our brain malfunctions, we cannot fully communicate and express ourselves.

The brain is similar to a mainframe computer. Each part of the brain holds and stores the memory and the design of our whole body. The brain processes and sorts through information at such a rapid pace, that it seems none of us could possibly keep up. We can, however, learn to slow down and track the flow of messages.

We can also learn how to communicate new messages through our brain and spinal cord down into any system or organ of the body. (Amen, 1998; Doidge, 2007)

Here are some questions to consider

...when you are working with your nervous system.

Imagine your nervous system transmitting security and safety coming from a deep flow of trust within you.

How would you feel?

When your body is filled with mistrust and fear, how does this get expressed through your nervous system?

Which of your organs does fear affect?

Can you allow trust to be transmitted from the brain and into each system and organ of your body?

Imagine unconditional love and acceptance bathing your brain and being transmitted down this superhighway into all areas of your body.

Does it get blocked along any pathway? If so, where?

Can you breathe deeply and allow the consciousness of love to flow into that area?

If not, what stops you?

Maybe it is an old pain, a negative thought, or self judgment that causes a traffic jam.

When you are out of order with self-respect, plagued by fear and self doubt, the superhighway may become jammed-up.

Do you respect your own feelings and thoughts and give them time for exploration, or do you override them?

Do you respect yourself in relationship with others?

Do you submit and comply, or bully others?

If so, how does this affect your nervous system?

Give yourself the opportunity to explore how you listen and speak through your nervous system.

Is the information highway clogged by mistrust, self-judgments, self-doubt, or unhealthy relationships?

Only you have the answers to these questions.

Self-Healing Meditation for
the Nervous System
Communication and Control

Bring the image of the nervous system into your awareness. Place your right hand on your lower belly to connect to your lower spine and nerves, and your left hand on your chest to connect to your brain, upper spine and nerves. Have a talk with your nervous system and tell it you completely support all it has done for you.

Notice if any areas feel hot, cold, tense or frenetic. Do you have any negative thoughts or emotions?

Notice how the energy is flowing between different areas of your brain, spinal cord and nerves. Imagine love saturating your brain and travelling down your spine into all your nerves. Allow the nerves to communicate with ease and grace, messages from the brain to the rest of the body, and from the rest of the body back to the brain.

Let your nervous system know that you have complete trust and confidence in its natural communication and controlling abilities to come into harmony and balance.

Relax and just let loving energy flow into your nervous system including every single nerve cell

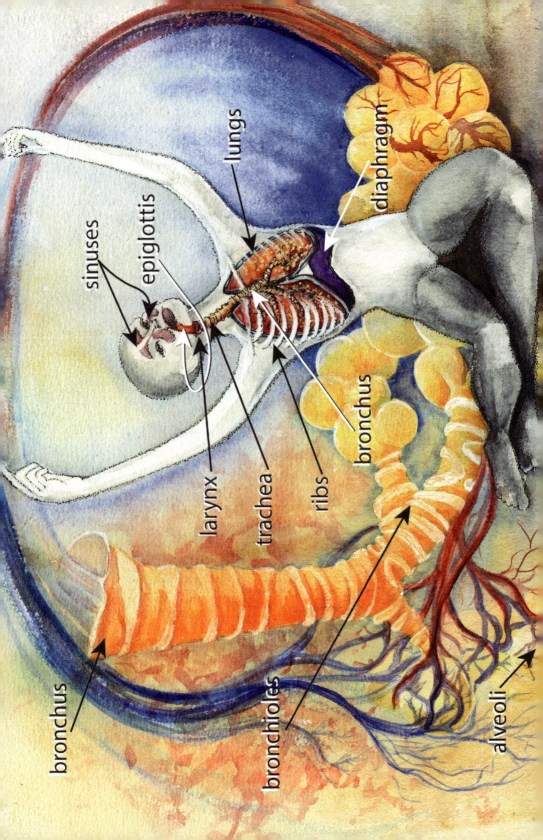

Chapter 3
The Respiratory System
Giving and Receiving Life

Each breath we take is life-giving. Our very first breath of life at our birthing immediately animates our physical body and marks the beginning of life as an independent human being. Then, upon our death when we take our last breath, our bodies are no longer animated and we are released once again to the source of unconditional love and universal oneness!

Anatomy and Physiology of the Respiratory System

The respiratory system works very closely with the heart and circulation system to support life and enhance our well-being. For example, our rhythmic breath helps synchronize the vibrations of the heartbeat throughout the body. The respiratory system, like all the other systems, is an integral part of the whole body. Its health both affects, and is dependent on, the health of the other parts of the whole.

> When we think about the respiratory system we tend to focus on the lungs, but the respiratory system is really so much more.

Breathing is both involuntary and voluntary. When we think about the respiratory system we tend to focus on the lungs, but the respiratory system is really so much more. Air first enters your body through your nose or mouth where it is moistened and warmed. The air then travels through your throat and voice box (larynx) and down through the windpipe (trachea and bronchus). The bronchus then splits into two tubes (called bronchi) that enter your lungs. Within the lungs, your bronchi branch into thousands of smaller, thinner tubes called bronchioles. These tubes end in bunches of tiny round air sacs called alveoli. Each of these air sacs is covered in a mesh of tiny blood vessels called capillaries. The capillaries connect to a network of arteries and veins through which the heart pumps blood throughout your body. It is in the alveoli that oxygen and carbon dioxide are exchanged. The respiratory system works with the circulatory system to support life by absorbing oxygen and releasing the waste product (carbon dioxide).

The respiratory muscles are essential to breathing and include the diaphragm, muscles between the ribs, abdominal muscles and some muscles in the neck and shoulder areas. Breathing is controlled by the nervous system and the rhythm of our breathing is naturally set. This natural setting varies in response to sensory information from the respiratory system and other parts of the body, and in response to concentrations of oxygen and carbon dioxide in the blood. Levels of oxygen and carbon dioxide in the blood lead to the stimulation of respiratory centres deep in the brain. Messages are then sent to the nervous system to increase or decrease breathing activity. For example, increased blood levels of carbon dioxide and decreased blood levels of oxygen increase the rate of breathing. Yet, within this intricate balancing act that directs automatic breathing, we can also voluntarily modify our breathing using the respiratory muscles innervated by this same nervous system. We do have control over our breathing. With this connection to the nervous system, we can intentionally influence the health of the body through breathing.

> *Our emotions are often reflected in the quality of our breath, often unbeknown to us..*

The Mind-Body Connection of the Respiratory System

The lungs bring in life-giving oxygen to the cells of the body; always receiving and then giving life with each breath. From a psycho-spiritual point of view, healthy breathing is seen to represent independence and a desire for life. Lung problems may suggest depression, grief, fear of life or not feeling worthy of living life fully. (Hay, 1998; Shapiro, 2006) Medical intuitive Carolyn Myss (1997) refers to the organs of the fourth chakra (heart and lungs) and how they can hold our grief, anger, and resentment. She also notes that the heart and lungs hold the energy and potential for forgiveness and compassion. Choa Kok Sui in his book *Advanced Pranic Healing* (1992), clearly outlines the energy centres that control and energize the respiratory system. These include the energy centre at the nose (sixth chakra), the throat (fifth chakra), the back heart (fourth chakra), and the solar plexus (third chakra). He goes on to explain how to work with these chakras to release emotional blockages to clear respiratory illness. Breathing not only maintains physical life, but it brings consciousness to the body. In the womb, the mother supplies the oxygen needed so the baby depends on her respiratory system and her breath while its own system develops. At birth, this beautiful system is activated the moment the infant is detached from its mother's umbilical cord. The baby's first breath is its first act of independence from its mother. The baby becomes animated and viable on its own. Then at death, the essence of life is released. If you have ever witnessed someone take their last breath, you may have felt their spirit or their life essence disappear at the same time.

Our breath is in constant flow and exchange with the air around us. It is a powerful system which can be used to affect our mental, spiritual and physical health. Our emotions are often reflected in the quality of our breath, sometimes unbeknown to us. On the other hand, we can transform how we feel simply by changing the pattern of our breathing voluntarily. For example, the rhythm of breathing has the ability to calm and focus the mind. Most meditation practices focus on the flow of breath. Breath work can also be used to work through pain in any part of the body.

> ...we can transform how we feel simply by changing the pattern of our breathing...

We often take this very simple process of breath for granted. It operates automatically beneath our consciousness.

Many times we are unaware of the process until we stop our breath, experience rapid breathing when feeling anxious or under stress, or perhaps when we meditate and learn to focus on our breath. There's great potential for healing here. You might unconsciously restrict your breathing, but you also have the ability to relax it. We may find ourselves saying things such as "I can't breathe," "I feel like I'm suffocating," or "I got the wind knocked out of me." When you're trying to calm someone down, what's the first thing you usually tell them to do? Take a deep breath. It's often the first thing we can rein in. We take that deep breath. We slow our breathing down. We come into the moment and can respond more calmly. A better sense of well-being usually follows. Here we have a powerful system that we can control and influence our mental, spiritual and physical health.

> *Here we have a powerful system that we can control to influence our mental, spiritual and physical health.*

Some questions to consider

...when working with your respiratory system.

Imagine how your breath flows when you experience trust, unconditional love and acceptance for yourself. Feel the ease and pleasure as self-love and self-acceptance flows from your breath.

How deeply do you breathe?

Does the air go all the way into your chest, or does it stop midway?

Now for a moment, imagine what mistrust, self-criticism and self-hate feels like as it flows with your breath throughout your body.

How do negative thoughts and emotions affect your breath?

How does the depth and rhythm of your breath change as your mood changes?

Mistrust can have a direct effect on your breath in different ways, such as shallow breathing, or anxious, rapid breathing.

Has trust and independence been eroded in your life?

Now, return your thoughts to unconditional love and acceptance, and notice if there is a change in your breath and how you feel.

You may also want to consider how your relationships affect how you breathe. For instance, when you are in harmony with someone, you feel at ease and the way you breathe reflects that easy feeling. On another occasion, you may meet someone and say, "They took my breath away." At other times, you may feel threatened or frightened by someone, and your breath either stops or becomes rapid and short.

Are there people in your life who are dominating or overbearing and interfere with your independence?

Are you in the way of yourself?

Do you feel smothered?

Do you smother yourself?

Do you find yourself frequently holding your breath?

Where Your Mind Goes Energy Flows – A Self-Healing Manual for the Mind and Body

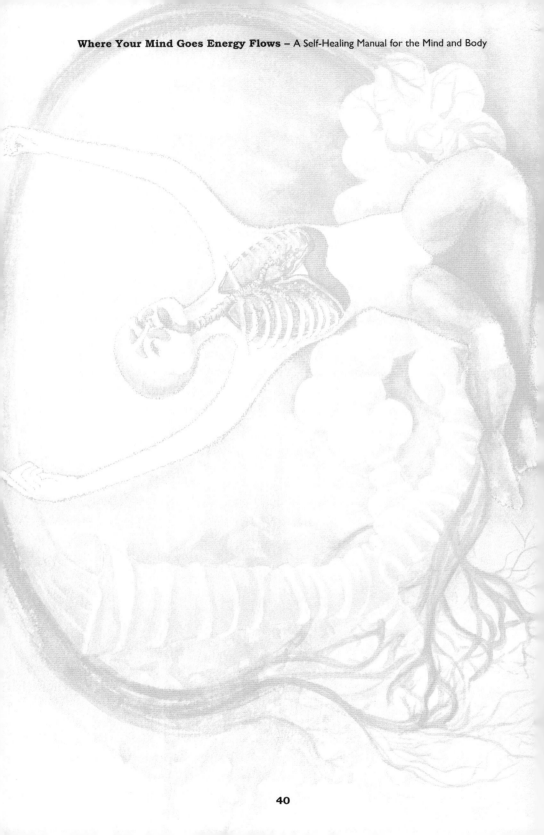

Self-Healing Meditation for the Respiratory System
Giving and Receiving Life

Bring the image of the airways and lungs into your awareness. Place your right hand on your lower belly to connect with the abdominal muscles for breathing, and your left hand on your chest to connect to your lungs, diaphragm and upper airways.

Connect with the rhythm of your breath and let it gently support you. Imagine if, with every breath you took, you made sure that it was laced with grace— the unconditional love of universal oneness. Imagine if the energy consciousness in these "Love Breaths" that you take then gets distributed to every single cell in your body.

Allow your breath to peacefully move and fill any empty, breathless places in your body. Trust that any problem areas will soften and dissipate on the winds of your breath. Relax and just let the gracefulness of each breath bring into harmony whatever is out of balance. Allow the purity of the respiratory system's ability to breathe in life easily and support the heart's mission of delivering love with grace to the whole body.

Trust in your respiratory system's divine intention to receive and give life.

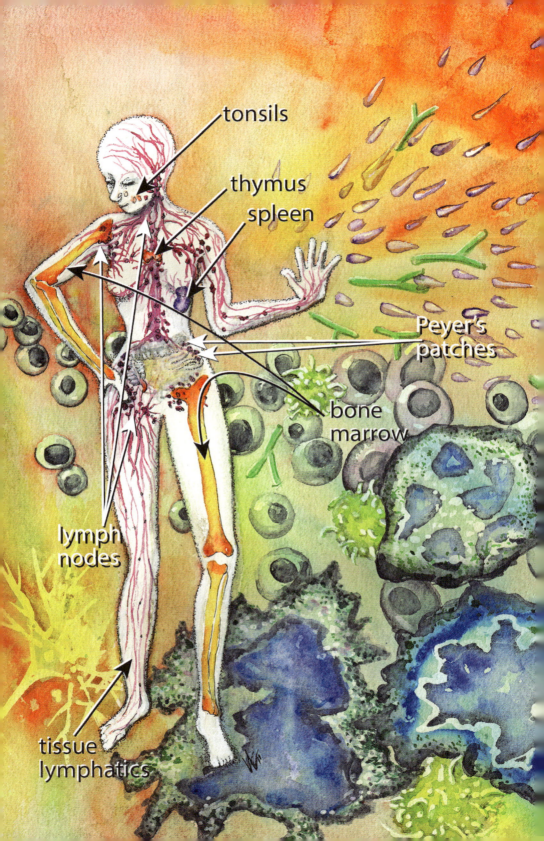

Chapter 4
The Immune System
Discernment and Protection

The immune system is your universal protective agent against harm and disease. It is wired for survival and is constantly learning, evolving, and working toward maintaining your health and well-being. The main intention of the immune system is to discern what is harmful to you and then to protect you against these harmful intrusions. These intruders may be as dangerous as a contagious virus, as complex as an abusive relationship, or as simple as a sliver in your finger.

Anatomy and Physiology of the Immune System

Some aspects of the immune system work locally and other immune responses are systemic and work throughout the body. A remarkable talent of the immune system is that it has a memory function, in that it can recognize intruders that have previously entered the body, and is able to create a stronger defence mechanism to deactivate the familiar intruder. At birth it is immature and cannot defend itself against all invaders. As we grow older and wiser in our ability to be discerning and to take care of ourselves, our immune system strengthens.

> A properly functioning immune system is able to discern between what is harmful and what is harmless.

A properly functioning immune system is able to discern between what is harmful and what is harmless. Once a harmful agent is detected in the body, the immune system puts into action an appropriate response to protect the body and eliminate the harmful intruder. When the immune system cannot discern what is harmful or is overwhelmed by outside invading substances or energies, it may not be able to protect and defend. An underactive immune system can lead to frequent or chronic illness; abnormal cell development may occur, such as in cancer. On the other hand, if the immune system is hyper-sensitive and becomes overactive it may give rise to autoimmune disorders like multiple sclerosis, chronic fatigue syndrome and some forms of arthritis and diabetes. There are also cases where the immune system responds inappropriately to harmless substances. This is the case with allergies.

White Blood Cells

The working cellular unit of the immune system is the white blood cell. White blood cells can move quickly and independently through the bloodstream, lymph system and through cell walls to where they are needed. There are several kinds of white blood cells, each having a different function in the complex process of immunity. These white blood cells come in various shapes and sizes and have specific tasks to defend and protect. For example, some destroy bacteria while others are designed to detect and attack cancer cells.

The Lymphatic System

The lymphatic system consists of vessels which are found throughout the body. These vessels connect the spleen, thymus, lymph nodes and other lymphoid tissues. Lymph fluid carrying white blood cells flows through these vessels to bathe all cells of the body, and clear out invaders, debris and toxins. White blood cells are also transported around the body through the bloodstream. The circulatory and lymphatic systems work together to protect the entire body.

Lymph nodes are small beanlike structures lying along the course of the lymphatic vessels. Large collections of nodes are found in the neck, groin, and armpits. Some are also found around the heart. Here in the lymph nodes, foreign or harmful substances are identified and deactivated by white blood cells like T and B cells. Some white blood cells make antibodies. Antibodies are special proteins that can trap and destroy disease causing agents.

Spleen and Lymphoid Tissues

The spleen is located in the upper left quadrant of the abdomen. Its role in the immune system is to filter blood and to detect and remove harmful invaders. It also plays a role in the production of antibodies and storage of white blood cells. The network of lymphoid tissues are found throughout the body including the digestive system, urogenital systems, respiratory system (including tonsils, nose and larynx) as well as in arteries, skin, the thyroid gland, salivary glands, breasts, and the eyes. Microorganisms and other harmful intruders that enter these areas will trigger an immune response to neutralize, destroy and remove them from the body. Peyer's patches are an example of such lymphoid tissues in the digestive system.

Bone Marrow and the Thymus Gland

Bone marrow and the thymus gland are involved in the creation and maturation of white blood cells. Red bone marrow lies deep within certain bones of the body: skull, ribs, breastbone, vertebrae, hipbones and the ends of long bones. All the white blood cells of the immune system are produced by stem cells in the red bone marrow. The thymus gland is found in the upper chest above the heart and behind the breastbone. It is here that white blood cells mature into T-cells. The thymus gland gradually enlarges during childhood until puberty. After puberty, the gland begins to shrink yet continues to function throughout life. The thymus gland is considered one of the major players in the immune system. At times of openness and happiness the T-cell count is high and it is more difficult to succumb to an illness. Con-

The immune system is not only discerning about what is harmful to us on a physical level but also on the emotional level of living.

versely, depression and loneliness is associated with a low T-cell count. (Shapiro, 2006)

The Mind-Body Connection of the Immune System

The immune system teaches us about how we care for ourselves, physically, psychologically, and spiritually. When it breaks down it relays clear messages that something has gone awry. It's only in recent years that the medical profession has come to recognize that there is a strong connection between emotions, negative thoughts, stress, and the health of the immune system. (Maté, 2004; Weil, 1998) The new field of psychoneuroimmunology suggests that emotional stress may be a significant influence in the health and effectiveness of the immune system. This means the system is affected by how we feel and think. The immune system is not only discerning about what is harmful to us on a physical level but also on the psychological level of living.

> *When we lose our sense of self we become open to invasion from outside forces.*

The immune system is governed by the energies of the second chakra which, when healthy, support feelings of self-love and acceptance. (Brennan, 1988) This system is very sensitive and can become overworked and weakened by chronic emotional stress such as abuse, grief, loss, anxiety and fear, real or imagined. (Maté, 2004) Conversely, with trust and love in flow, one can more easily identify what is harmful without being overly influenced by outside forces. Being grounded in our own thoughts, feelings, and individuality offers us the opportunity to discern whether or not to internalize external influences we encounter in our lives. If we mindlessly submit our power to another person, group, ideology or culture for example, we lose our identity and become vulnerable on many levels. When we lose our sense of self we become open to

> *...our ability to have boundaries is essential to our health and well-being.*

invasion from outside forces. On a physical and psychological level, our ability to have boundaries is essential to our health and well-being. (Shapiro, 2006)

Here are some questions to consider

...when you are working with your immune system.

Do you live on high alert? Are you overly stressed, depressed or worried?

Have you ever lost your sense of individuality or confidence in your own beliefs?

All of this can deplete your sense of trust in life and interfere with the health of your immune system. An overactive immune system may indicate a habit of self-loathing and disrespect of self. Ask yourself if you are becoming increasingly intolerant and irritable with others or yourself.

Can you open up to self-love and acceptance for all of who you are, just the way you are?

Would it be possible to let this self-loving consciousness flow into your immune system; to allow the natural function of discernment and protection to unfold on your behalf?

Standing in one's power and being autonomous is not always easy. As life unfolds, it can serve up a vast array of pressures and influences which complicate our emotional existence. Knowing where you stand and where you belong—in your family, with your friends, and at work—helps build a sense of self-respect.

How are you at respecting yourself?

Have you been unduly influenced by someone or something else?

Is there a physical or emotional part of you that you have been ignoring or denying?

Do you have to work hard to maintain your sense of self?

Do you step out of your integrity in your interpersonal relationships to gain favour?

Relationships that support you and reflect your unique gifts and qualities back to you, help to nourish your emotional health and thus the health of the immune system.

Self-Healing Meditation for **the Immune System**

Discernment and Protection

Bring the image of the immune system into your awareness. Place your right hand on your lower belly to connect to your spleen, lymph nodes, and bone marrow of the lower body, and place your left hand on your chest to connect to the thymus gland, the bone marrow and lymph nodes of the upper body.

Let loving energy flow from your hands, calling on every white blood cell within the body to discern any disease activity and know when to mobilize efforts to deactivate it.

Notice where you feel vulnerable and don't know how to protect yourself. Notice if there are any areas of loneliness, grief, sadness, fear or anger in your body. Allow these areas to be bathed in self-love and acceptance.

With trust in flow, you can more easily identify what is getting in the way or what is harmful, without being overly influenced by outside forces.

Let the immune system's natural discerning and protective forces come into harmony and balance.

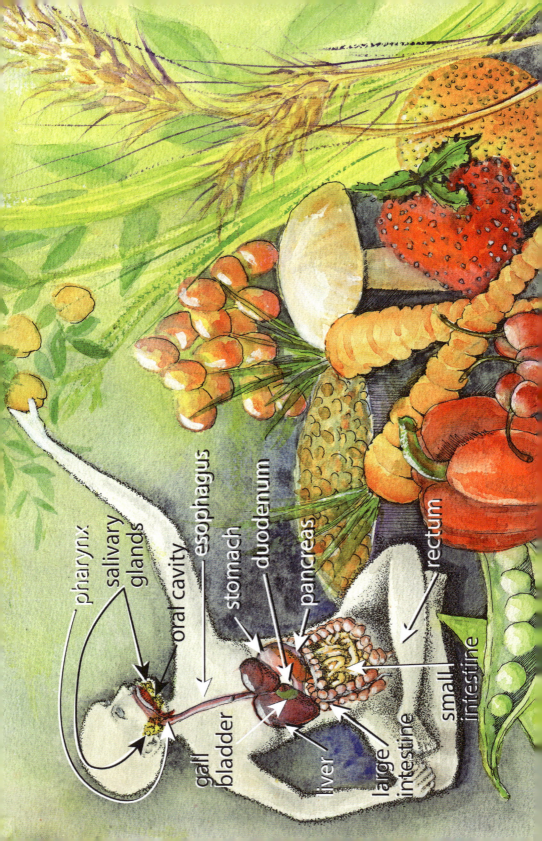

Chapter 5
The Digestive System
Nourishment and Contentment

Many of us go through life eating what we want, when we want, without any knowledge of how our digestive system functions. Furthermore, from infancy into adulthood our digestive system can change dramatically. Foods that we digested in early childhood can cause major problems later on in life. A balanced nutritious diet affects all the other body systems and thus is perhaps the most essential daily contribution to our health.

Anatomy and Physiology of the Digestive System

This system is vital to our well-being. We survive on all it digests and we depend on it to eliminate what is not useful to us. The process of digestion involves the breaking down of food into a form that can be absorbed and used by the body. Once the food enters the mouth, it travels through the esophagus, stomach, small intestine and colon (or large intestine) before the wastes are excreted through the rectum and anus. A series of contractions by the smooth muscle lining of the digestive tract helps move the food and wastes along through the system. There are a few other organs involved as well; the liver, pancreas and gall bladder all help the body to break down, absorb and utilize food. The interesting thing is that this process doesn't work in exactly the same way

> *The process of digestion involves the breaking down of food into a form that can be absorbed and used by the body.*

for everyone. We each have different amounts of acids and enzymes within us. We break down food differently. We have different sensitivities to different foods. In addition, the digestive system is very susceptible to emotional stress which vary from person to person.

Digestion of food begins the moment we place food in our mouths. Chewing food and mixing it with saliva breaks it down into smaller particles so it can be digested. Saliva is also produced in the mouth to prevent bacterial infections, lubricate the mouth and food, and to begin the breakdown of starches and fats. Saliva contains the enzymes to break down starches and fats. In our busy society, we tend to eat too quickly and not chew our food thoroughly enough. This can increase the burden on the digestive organs because they have to work harder to break down the poorly chewed food. Experts on digestion say we should chew each mouthful of food 35 times! The food then moves from the mouth through the esophagus to the stomach. Our stomach churns the food, mixing it with enzymes that help digest proteins, fat, vitamins, and minerals. Stomach enzymes include various substances, like stomach acid, necessary for digestion to occur. When stomach acid levels are out of balance we can experience problems such as acid reflux or gas.

As the food moves on to the small intestine, enzymes from the pancreas and small intestine are released to digest and absorb carbohydrates, fats, and proteins. Bile salts secreted from the gallbladder also help with the digestion and absorption of fats and nutrients such as vitamins A, D, E, and K. The pancreas produces and secretes several enzymes and hormones involved in continuing the digestion of carbohydrates, fats and protein. The hormones it secretes, one of which is insulin, are responsible for controlling sugar metabolism. When the pancreas cannot produce enough insulin, the condition called diabetes develops. The liver regulates the composition of circulating blood by filtering all the blood that leaves the lining of the digestive tract. It stabilizes blood sugar and fat levels, removes excess proteins and wastes from the bloodstream, and stores vitamins and minerals. Finally, the liver secretes bile into the gallbladder, where it is stored until it is excreted into the small intestine to emulsify and break down fats. The liver is a very busy organ.

The small intestines are nestled together within the abdomen and the large intestine is curled around them. Most of the digestion and the absorption of food nutrients occurs in the first portion of the small intestines. Here too, enzymes and hormones assist with digestion and absorption. By the time food reaches the colon or large intestine, most of the nutrients have been absorbed, leaving indigestible fibre and water. The leftover solids are stored and compacted as they move down through the length of the large intestine. The large intestine re-absorbs water, electrolytes, and a few vitamins back into the body and then sends the rest out for elimination.

The Mind-Body Connection of the Digestive System

> ...the digestive process is not just about taking in food to fuel the body, it is very much linked to social and emotional needs...

The digestive system performs a vital and complex function to the health and well-being of our bodies. Even more though, food and eating play an important and integral role in our lives every day. Food shopping and cooking is usually a daily activity. Meals are often the time when we gather together with family and friends.

From a holistic perspective, the digestive process is not just about taking in food to fuel the body; it is very much linked to social and emotional needs like comfort, love and belonging. We know that emotional factors can influence the functioning of the system. For example, it is well known now that stomach ulcers are exacerbated by stress. Other digestion problems may well be linked to stress from work, family or friends. If we grew up with abuse or live with an angry partner, we may feel that we have to "swallow" negative emotions for fear of more abuse. We may have undigested anger boiling inside of us, which interferes with our ability to relax and digest our food easily at meal time. It has been suggested that stomach problems including indigestion are associated with fear, problems with self esteem and self-respect, lack of self care, difficulty with decision making, and sensitivity to criticism. (Shapiro, 2006; Hay, 1998; Myss, 1997).

From birth we are focused on food. We cry and are rewarded by warm milk and mother's love and attention. In these early years we do not how to separate food, parents and love. This continues to be a focus of our happiness or frustration, depending on our experiences as the years go on. Eating continues to be one of the most emotional and controversial activities throughout one's life. What we eat, how we eat, when we eat, why we eat, all varies from one person to the next and many of us are attached to our eating habits. Food may be a substitute for love and may be used as a punishment through deprivation. Our relationship to food and eating is not simple. It affects our physical, emotional and spiritual health.

Often people find themselves turning to food when bored, angry, depressed or nervous. Just as you may try to fill an inner emptiness with food, so you may reject or deny your needs and therefore reject food. Indigestion is strongly associated with worry and anxiety. It is here in the stomach that we tend to harbour worry as the digestive juices churn with anxiety. Constipation may well become a way to control life by holding onto things and resisting change. Letting go may bring feelings of powerlessness. On the other hand, diarrhea may occur due to feelings of fear and anxiety when one is overwhelmed by emotions and unable to assimilate and process what is going on in life. (Shapiro, 2006; Hay, 1998)

> *Indigestion and other digestive problems are often the first physical signs of stress and life's difficulties.*

It is interesting to note, that there are two main chakras that supply energy to the digestive system. The third chakra governs the consciousness of one's place in the universe and intentionality toward health. The fifth chakra governs the expression of self, ability to ask for needs, and ability to receive. (Brennan, 1988) Digestion is closely connected to the third chakra and the associated psycho-spiritual needs of self-respect and personal power. Those who are obese often remark they have "no control" when it comes to food and those with anorexia nervosa exercise massive amounts of control over their intake of food often to the point of serious physical health problems and even death. Shapiro (2006) suggests that "With anorexia nervosa there is a denying of yourself and an unconscious longing to disappear, as if by becoming small your needs and presence also diminish, especially your need to be loved." (p. 244)

With obesity, the excess weight can become an illusionary buffer between our inner selves and the fearful outside world. Unfortunately, the weight can also block out access to our own feelings leaving us feeling empty and alone. In Dr. Northrup's book (2003) *The Wisdom of Menopause*, she claims that "Women with substantial weight problems usually have unresolved issues in the third emotional centre. The health of the third emotional centre depends on a balance between responsibility to ourselves and responsibility to others, and also on our sense of self esteem" (p. 221).

As we can see, the digestive system is a monitor of our emotional balance. Indigestion and other digestive problems are often the first physical signs of stress and life's difficulties. When we are happy our digestive system is usually maintenance free.

Here are some questions to consider

...when you are working with your digestive system.

What has gotten in the way of your ability to receive love and affection to nourish your inner self?

What life situations are difficult to "swallow" in your life?

How has trust in receiving the love you deserve been eroded?

What childhood traumas have deteriorated your ability to know what is nourishing to you?

We often question or doubt ourselves, we're either unsure which foods are best for us, or we don't pay attention to the foods we consume. As trust in your ability to nourish yourself grows, you can more naturally choose foods that make you feel good and eat just enough, in a more relaxed way.

Do you have difficulty assimilating aspects of your life into reality?

Are you having trouble processing stress and unhappy events in your life?

As you deepen your awareness of how your digestive system functions and how intimately it is connected with your physical and emotional health, you will be more able to take charge of your well being.

Self-Healing Meditation for the Digestive System
Nourishment and Contentment

Bring the image of the digestive system into your awareness. Place your right hand on your lower belly to connect to your intestines, and the left hand just below your ribcage to connect to your stomach and upper digestive system.

Let energy flow to the small and large intestines in the lower abdomen and into the stomach radiating up through to the mouth and down to the liver, gall bladder, and pancreas to relax and soothe any disorder of the digestive and elimination system of the body. Track the energy consciousness and notice if any images or feelings emerge.

Relax and let love and nourishment flow to your whole digestive system. Allow this system to help you choose nourishing foods that are right for you. Let the gracefulness of your digestion and ease of elimination come into balance and harmony.

Trust in your digestive system's intention to bring nourishment and contentment to your life.

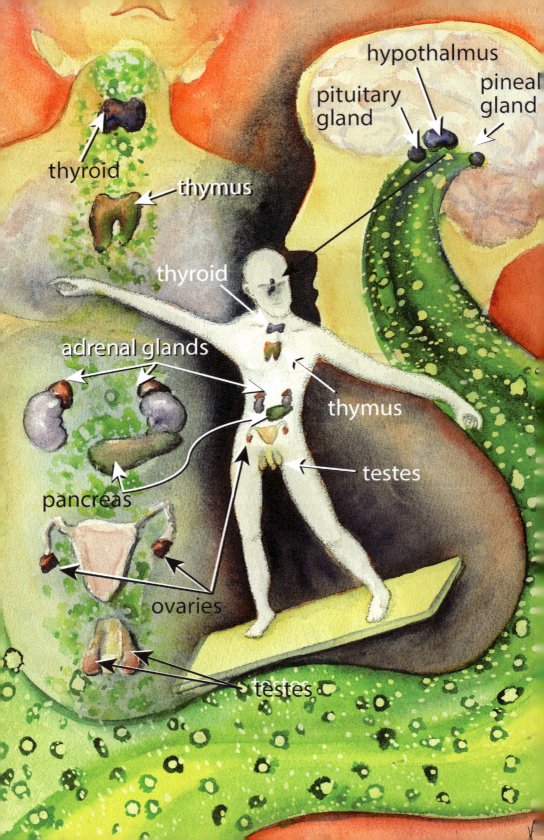

Chapter 6

The Endocrine System

Balance and Coordination

The endocrine system is incredibly complex involving many different organs, substances and cells organized into specific structures throughout the body. In cooperation with other body systems, the endocrine system helps with balancing and coordinating the body's many functions. It accomplishes these vital tasks through hormones produced and secreted from a network of glands and organs. Let's take a closer look at this system.

Anatomy and Physiology of the Endocrine System

The endocrine system is one of the body's main systems for communicating, controlling and coordinating the body's work. It has an innate wisdom that keeps the communication paced, clear and accurate, as it interacts and directly works with many other systems in the body. It works in concert with the nervous system, reproductive system, kidneys, gut, liver, pancreas and fat stores to help maintain and control energy levels, reproduction, growth and development, and *homeostasis*[1].

---

1   American Psychological Association (APA): homeostasis. (n.d.). Dictionary.com Unabridged. Retrieved November 3, 2017 from Dictionary.com website http://www.dictionary.com/browse/homeostasis
> *[hoh-mee-uh-stey-sis] noun, the tendency of a system, especially the physiological system of higher animals, to maintain internal stability, owing to the coordinated response of its parts to any situation or stimulus that would tend to disturb its normal condition or function.*

The endocrine system also helps the body respond appropriately to its environment, as well as to stress and injury. It accomplishes these vital tasks via a network of glands and organs that produce, store, and secrete certain types of hormones. Hormones are special chemicals that are made by cells and cause different effects on other cells, tissues or organs of the body. Hormones are delivered where they are needed through the bloodstream. Some hormones are released cyclically based on certain time patterns that often fit with daily body rhythms, like the sleep-wake cycle. A gland will stop secreting hormones when the level in the blood system has reached the amount needed. Through this steady feedback system, hormone imbalances are avoided.

Pituitary Gland

The pituitary gland, despite being pea sized, is often referred to as the "master gland" because of the many hormones it produces which influence several body systems. For example, these hormones help coordinate the reproductive functions in women and men, physical growth and development, water balance, and are involved in the stress response, just to name a few.

Hypothalamus

The hypothalamus occupies an area of the brain above the pituitary gland and acts as a connection between the nervous system and the endocrine system. It assists in the proper functioning of the pituitary gland and adrenal glands.

Pineal Gland

Scientists are still learning how the pineal gland works. They have found one hormone so far, called melatonin, that is produced by this gland. Melatonin may inhibit reproductive functions, protect against the damage that free radicals can cause, and set circadian rhythms including eating habits, sleep patterns and mood cycles.

Thyroid

The thyroid is a small butterfly shaped gland inside the neck, straddling the breathing airway (trachea) sitting below the Adam's apple. The thyroid hormones control the body's rate of metabolism. The hormone calcitonin is also secreted here, which inhibits the loss of calcium from the bones.

Parathyroid

The parathyroid gland consists of four small glands located behind the thyroid gland. They make hormones that help control calcium and phosphorous levels in the body. These are necessary for proper bone development, nerve conduction and muscle contraction.

Thymus

The thymus gland, as we have seen in our reviews of the immune system, is a gland needed especially early in life for normal immune function. The thymus gland secretes hormones called thymosins that target cells to help mature, coordinate and regulate the immune response.

Adrenal Glands

The adrenal glands are pyramid shaped. The outer portion is called the adrenal cortex and secretes hormones that help the body control blood sugar, increase the burning of protein and fat, decrease inflammation, and respond to stresses like fevers, major illnesses, and injuries. One of these hormones helps to control blood volume which can regulate blood pressure. The inner portion called the adrenal medulla produces hormones such as adrenalin, which are released during the stress response. These hormones control stress responses that result in increased blood glucose levels, increased heart rate and blood pressure, airway expansion to improve oxygen intake, and increased blood flow to muscles.

Pancreas

The pancreas has digestive and endocrine functions. The endocrine function of the pancreas consists of small groups of cells called the Islets of Langerhans. They secrete insulin and glucagon which maintain healthy blood sugar levels. This process is disrupted in the condition called diabetes.

Ovaries

The ovaries produce estrogen and progesterone. These hormones are responsible for developing and maintaining female sexual traits, regulating the menstrual cycle, as well as maintaining a pregnancy. The most common change in the production of ovarian hormones is caused by the start of menopause, which is part of the normal aging process. Menopause also occurs when ovaries are removed surgically.

Testes

The testes produce androgens (the main one being testosterone). During puberty, testosterone helps to bring about the physical changes that young boys experience as their bodies take on adult male characteristics. Throughout adult life, testosterone helps maintain the sex drive, sperm production, male hair patterns, muscle mass, and bone mass.

Additional organs that secrete hormones as part of their functional role in the body include the intestines, kidneys, heart, bones and adipose (fat) tissue.

The Mind-Body Connection of the Endocrine System

The endocrine system is charged with communicating, controlling and co-

> *With sophisticated emotional, neurological, hormonal and chemical feedback systems in place, the endocrine system helps to even out our energy levels needed for everyday life...*

ordinating many vital bodily functions and it works directly with many other body systems. It helps control and coordinate balance through all the ups and downs of the mind and body. The endocrine system, to work well, must be good at networking and needs partners that are willing to work together to get the job done—each doing their respective jobs faithfully. The endocrine system has structures situated throughout the body. Each of the seven major chakras influence a part of the endocrine system. This system has a part to play in all of the psycho-emotional aspects of being. (Eden; 1998, Myss, 1997; Brennan, 1988; Dale, 2009) "Chakras govern the endocrine system, so bringing your chakras into balance brings your hormones, and thus your emotions, into balance as well." (Eden, 1998, p. 166) With sophisticated emotional, neurological, hormonal and chemical feedback systems in place, the endocrine system helps to even out our energy levels needed for everyday life in the face of the many stresses and traumas we suffer. It works very closely with the nervous and circulatory systems both of which also play a major role in communication throughout the body. It is also very adept at reading the demands of our external environment. This system plays a huge role with reproduction and growth and development of the human species—keeping the family tree in business.

> *Imagine living with a steady and balanced sense of self-love and acceptance through the bumps of life at home and work. It would be like being your own best friend through thick and thin!*

The endocrine system responds to the changes in our physical and mental state of being. It innately knows how to do this. It has an intimate connection with all that is happening through its feedback systems. It easily networks with other parts of the body and mind to bring about healthy patterns of being in all aspects of life. Imagine how living with mistrust and fear could interrupt the work of this beautifully coordinated system. Imagine how a life full of one crisis after the next would be very taxing to a system responsible for maintaining balance. Imagine living with a steady and balanced sense of self-love and acceptance through the bumps of life at home and work. It would be like being your own best friend through thick and thin! Your endocrine system holds this steadiness and brings us back to homeostasis through the undulations of life.

Questions to consider

...when working with your endocrine system.

Ask yourself how you are at keeping balanced & coordinating your life tasks.

How does being balanced feel to you? Does it feel foreign to you?

Do you thrive on crisis and the extremes of living?

Can you relax and trust in a steady, balanced way of life?

Do you see yourself as unbalanced and unable to right yourself after a crisis?

Can you see yourself moving through life changes easily?

When you were growing up, was your family able to operate in a balanced and coordinated way most of the time? Or, did you feel life was always falling apart?

Do you have difficulty working harmoniously with others?

How are you at networking and communicating with family, friends, and at work?

Do you have difficulty delivering messages accurately?

Do you respect the hormonal fluctuations in your body?

How was puberty for you?

Did you feel respected by the people in your life as you went through puberty?

If you are in menopause, what are your feelings about your hormonal activities changing?

Reflect for a moment, fully trusting that life can unfold in a balanced and coordinated fashion. Imagine that as problems arise, your body and mind quickly respond in ways that bring you back into an even balanced flow once again.

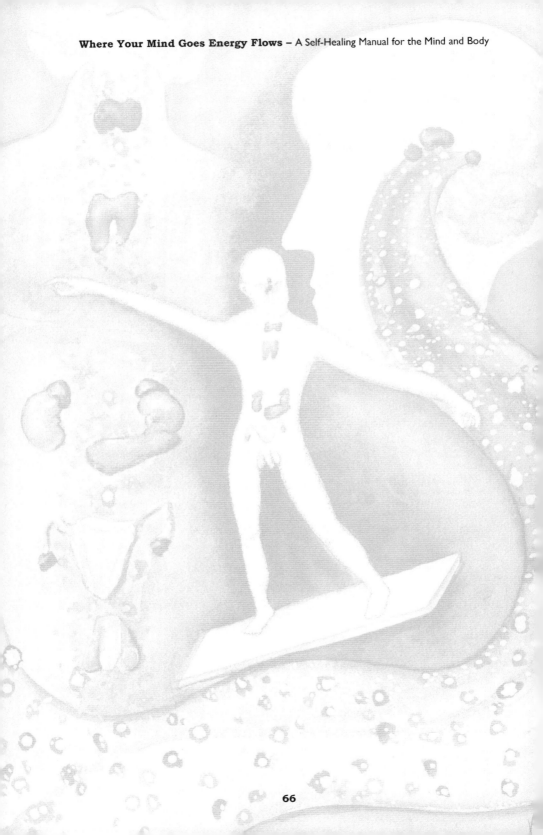

Self-Healing Meditation for the Endocrine System
Balance and Coordination

Bring the image of the endocrine system to your awareness. Place your right hand on your lower belly to connect to the adrenals, pancreas and gonads, and the left hand on your chest to connect with the thymus gland, thyroid and parathyroid glands. Later, you can also move your left hand to gently hold the bridge of your nose to connect with the pituitary, pineal and hypothalamus glands.

Take a deep breath. Relax and allow energy to flow into your endocrine system. Notice if any areas are blocked and wait there until the energy starts to move again. Simply trust in the endocrine system's unique and amazing ability to balance out the ups and downs of life.

Let everything go as you unfold into a peaceful state of relaxation.

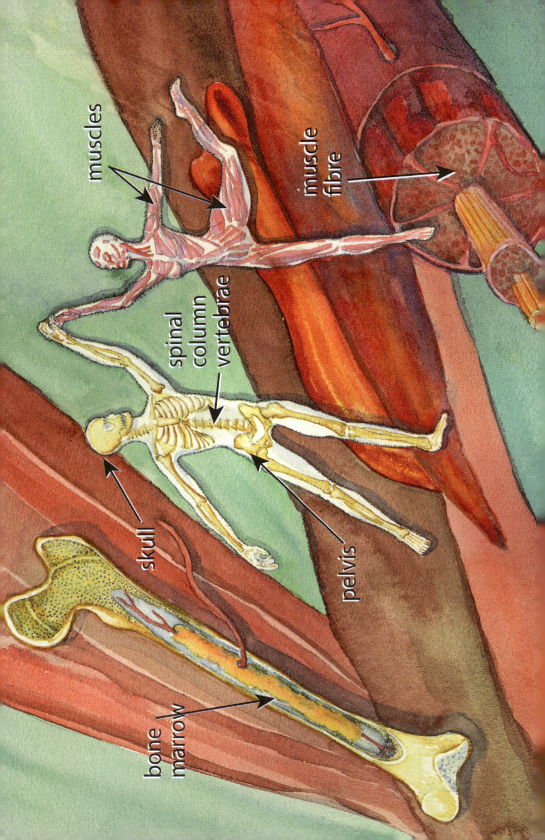

Chapter 7
The Musculoskeletal System
Support and Mobility

The musculoskeletal system is often referred to as the locomotor system. However, it provides more than just locomotion. It provides the body with exquisite support, stability, protection and shape. The bones are involved in the production of blood cells and storage of essential minerals. It is such an ingenious body system with all the abilities to provide for smooth, graceful, flexible mobility, protection and stability.

Anatomy and Physiology of the Musculoskeletal System

The musculoskeletal system consists of the body's bones (the skeleton), muscles, cartilage, tendons, ligaments, joints, and other connective tissue. Connective tissue is the tissue that supports and binds tissues and organs together. The musculoskeletal system's primary functions include supporting the body, allowing motion, and protecting vital organs. In addition, the skeletal portion of this system serves as the main storage system for calcium and phosphorus, and contains critical components for the formation of blood cells.

Bones are connected to other bones and muscle fibres via connective tissues such as tendons and ligaments. The bones provide stable framework to our bodies. Muscles keep our bones in place and also play a role in movement of the bones. To further allow motion, bones are connected by joints. Cartilage within the joint prevent the bone ends from rubbing directly on to each other. Muscles contract to move the bone attached at the joint.

The Skeletal System

Strong yet light, the skeletal system is made of living bone material with networks of blood vessels running throughout. Bones are hard and rigid on the outside and softer on the inside. An average adult skeleton consists of 206 bones and accounts for about twenty percent of the total body weight. The skeletal system serves the body to provide shape, support, stability, movement, storage of minerals, blood cell production, and protection of inner organs like the brain and heart. The red marrow of some bones is the site for blood cell production. Approximately 2.6 million red blood cells are created per second in order to replace existing cells that have been destroyed by the liver as part of their normal life cycle. The dynamic storage system in the bones is important because it helps regulate the balance of minerals such as calcium and phosphorous in the bloodstream.

Muscles, Connective Tissues and Joints

The human body consists of about seven hundred muscles, of which there are three types; cardiac, smooth, and skeletal. Cardiac and smooth muscles are not considered a part of the musculoskeletal system. Cardiac muscles are found in the heart and are used only to circulate blood. Smooth muscles are used to control the flow of substances within the passageways of hollow organs like our intestines. Smooth and cardiac muscles are not under conscious control. Skeletal muscles are mostly under conscious control as they are the muscles we use to move the bones of our body. Skeletal muscles are attached to bones and arranged in opposing groups around joints. Muscles are innervated by nerves, which conduct electrical currents from the nervous system and cause the muscles to contract, which in turn, move the bones.

Connective tissue also provides structure, protecting and supporting most parts of the body. Fascia is the soft component of the connective tissue. Tendons and ligaments, known as deep fascia, make up the strongest form of connective tissue. Tendons are tough, flexible bands of fibrous tissue that connect muscles to bones. As muscles contract, tendons transmit the force to the rigid bones, pulling on them and causing movement. Ligaments are small bands of dense, white, fibrous and elastic tissue. They connect the ends of bones together in order to form a joint. Most ligaments limit dislocation, or prevent certain movements that may cause breaks.

Joints connect individual bones and help them move against each other. The various joints allow for a great variety of motion, and the function of each joint is closely related to its structure. When movement is not required, such as between the bones of the skull, the joint is immobile and strong. These bones are locked together as if they were a single bone. Joints between the vertebrae (back bone), allow limited movement while still maintaining a certain amount of strength. In areas where movement is more important than strength, joints are freely movable. The shoulder joint, for example, allows the arm to move in a variety of ways. Because it allows such a range of motion, the shoulder joint is relatively weak and prone to injury.

> *A beautiful marriage of yin and yang is playing out within the musculoskeletal system.*
>
> *Our yin energy is fluid through the flexibility of the system and our yang energy is held beautifully in the firm structure of the system.*

The Mind-Body Connection of the Musculoskeletal System

The musculoskeletal system's intention is to provide integrity, support, protection, movement and expression. The soft bone marrow within nourishes the body with minerals and salts. It creates white blood cells for immunity and red blood cells for vitality. The hard dense bone gives us strength and stability, while the muscles give us flexibility and animate our whole being. A beautiful marriage of yin and yang is playing out within the musculoskeletal system. Our yin energy is fluid through the flexibility of the system and our yang energy is held beautifully in the firm structure of the system.

Our posture and how we walk or move can communicate to others how we are feeling and what we are thinking. We often call this "body language." The musculoskeletal system creates the framework in which we live, and allows for movement and expression of our thoughts, beliefs, ideas and feelings. The more fluid and flexible the system is, the more fluid and flexible our expression and movement will be. Our emotions affect our body movements and in turn, our body movements can affect our emotions. Exercise is known to elevate our spirits, while lethargy can lead to depression. It is such a dynamic system.

> *Our emotions affect our body movements and in turn, our body movements can affect our emotions.*

Our bones are the framework of our existence. We can live with shrunken weak muscle tissue but we cannot live without strong bones. Our bones are the foundation of our physical being, just like one's family and home can form the foundation for a healthy social and emotional life. "Just as the bones support your physical being and give life to the muscles and fluids, so your core beliefs give you constant inner strength and support, while finding your expression in your lifestyle, behaviour, and relationships. Problems with your bones, therefore, represent conflict within the very core of your being." (Shapiro, 2006, p. 138)

> *Within the essence of bone, there is a deep quiet that effortlessly holds the vastness of our core being.*

Our skeletal structure and muscular mobility provide us with independence and a structural command of our space. Issues of the first chakra, like trust, safety, belonging and security, are connected to the hard tissue of bone. Within the essence of bone, there is a deep quiet that effortlessly holds the vastness of our core being. If you have ever broken a bone, especially in a limb, perhaps you experienced deep fears of vulnerability. It can affect one down to the core, as if one's support system has been pulled out from under them. One's foundation is rattled.

Life issues and traumas, repressed anxieties, doubts of self worth, as well as joy and love are reflected in the condition of our organs, flesh, and especially our muscles. Our muscles hold and can release tension from traumas and negative feelings. When we are unable to release stress and tension, this gradual buildup is stored in the muscles and connective tissue leaving us fixed in a restricted form. We can create shields of armour with the fascia to hold back emotions such as fear, anger, or grief. A particular emotional veil can be built into the muscular system locking in the associated mental attitude. For example, rigidity of the musculoskeletal system can suggest problems with being flexible in life, holding anger and resentment, being resistant to change, and feeling unsupported in life. (Hay, 1998) Some healing practices focus solely on releasing tension in the connective tissues. They are based on the knowing that the body's connective tissues can store emotional trauma. A healthy dynamic musculoskeletal system enables all body systems such as the circulatory, digestive, respiratory, immune and nervous systems to function properly. Tension in the muscles will affect all the other body systems.

Personal growth requires addressing our issues from both the mind and body perspectives. If our core beliefs about support, flexibility and security are densely held in the musculoskeletal system, and if we bring more conscious awareness to our bones and muscles, perhaps we can shift our thoughts toward more positive and unifying belief systems.

Questions to consider

...when working with your musculoskeletal system.

It would benefit us greatly if we could mindfully listen to what our bones and muscles need.

> *Do your muscles feel flexible?*
>
> *Where do you feel tense?*
>
> *Do you feel deep-seated anger or fear in your body?*
>
> *How would you dance if no one was watching?*
>
> *What movements would you want to make?*

Imagine if your core beliefs were sourced from a place of solid self-respect?

> *Do your bones feel strong?*
>
> *Do your beliefs feel strong?*
>
> *Do you have any core issues within yourself that are in conflict?*
>
> *What are you aching for?*

Imagine the powerful being that you are, with a strong, supportive skeletal structure and fluid, mobile muscles. Empowerment comes from deep within the core of your being held in your bones. Self-empowerment can be expressed through your physical body.

Look at your hands and imagine seeing deeply into the bones and muscles.

> *What do you see?*
>
> *What core beliefs are being reflected back to you from the shape of your fingers or way you hold your hands?*

Now picture your spine, your shoulders, your legs or your feet.

> *What do you see here?*

Allowing yourself to play with a deepened sense of sight can deepen your connection to what is being held in the consciousness of your body structures.

Have you ever felt that you knew, deep in your bones, the truth of what caused a certain situation or crisis?

Often we hear people say, "I can feel it in my bones." Imagine if we could open up more consciously to this intuitive wisdom that is held deeply in the framework of our bodies.

Have you ever watched a dance performance and been deeply touched emotionally? Did you completely understand the message the dancer was communicating, all without words?

Imagine if you could allow the light of pure love to anoint your bones and muscles with the freedom of expression.

Could this help you communicate truths about yourself?

Could this open up avenues for growth and transformation?

How do you physically express yourself?

When you greet someone do you automatically make certain movements or body gestures?

Do your body gestures match what you are verbally communicating?

Do some relationships make your muscles or bones feel weak or strong?

Bring your awareness to your physical activities, such as your normal way of walking, the way you usually sit, or how you embrace another person. This heightened awareness may help you learn what is going on deep within the core of your being.

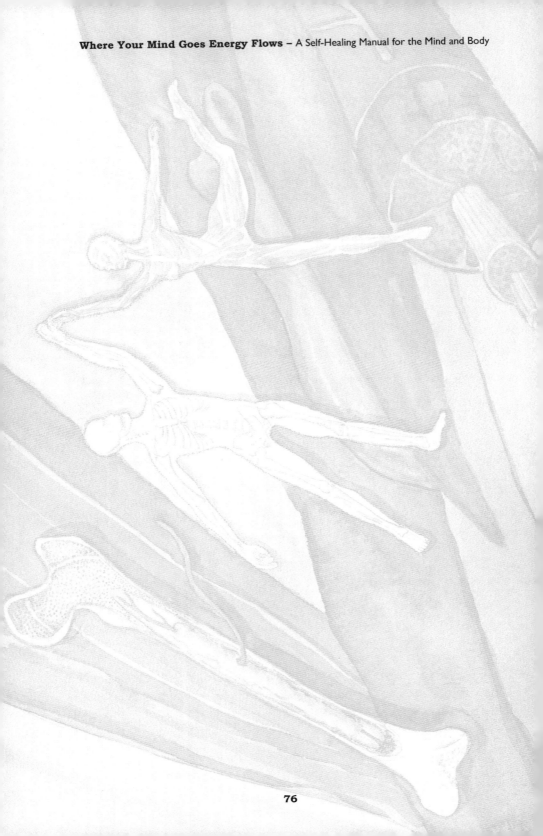

Self-Healing Meditation for
the Musculoskeletal System
Support and Mobility

Bring the image of the musculoskeletal system to your awareness. Place your right hand on your lower belly and your left hand on your breastbone to connect deeply into your muscles and bones.

Breathe deeply. Relax and let the energy flow lovingly into your muscles, ligaments, tendons, fascia and bones. Sink deeply into the essence of your bones and connect to your deepest longings.

Notice any core beliefs about life emerging. Let the healing energy flow into any areas that are giving you problems until they come into relaxation and peace.

Allow feelings of support, flexibility and freedom of physical expression upwell into your whole being.

Support the primary intention of your bones and muscles of all kinds to protect, support, and give structural integrity and mobility to the body with harmony and balance.

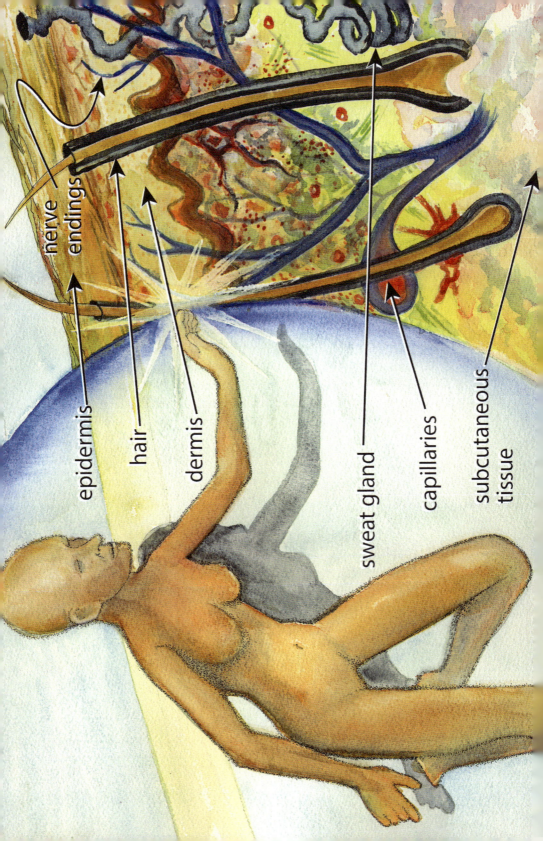

Chapter 8

The Skin System

Boundary of Reception and Protection

Our skin is incredibly flexible and multitalented. The skin is the largest organ of the body and accomplishes many incredible functions. The skin is waterproof, yet able to release water. It protects the inner body from infections and injury, yet is extremely sensitive to touch, heat, cold and pain. It is our first line of defence against nature's elements as it forms a protective layer around the entire surface of the body. It is completely washable, self-mending and regulates our body temperature. We cannot live comfortably without healthy skin. How does the skin accomplish all this?

Anatomy and Physiology of the Skin

Our skin is the ultimate boundary between ourselves and the outside world. It is our skin that is upfront as we face others and our environment. It is our first line of reception and our first line of protection. On average the skin of an adult is about two square metres large depending on one's weight, height and size. The skin is one component of the body system which also includes nails, hair, sweat glands, and sebaceous (oil) glands. The skin, even though it appears to be thin, is made up of three layers. Each layer has its own function. The health of the skin reflects and depends on the health and activity of other body systems. For example, how well we digest food affects the health of the skin. Skin

> *It is our first line of reception and our first line of protection.*

is also affected by allergic reactions which are activated by the immune system.

The epidermis is the visible, topmost layer of the skin. This layer of skin is made up mostly of cells called keratinocytes. These cells contain keratin which is a type of insoluble fibrous protein that helps protect the body. Hair and nails are made of specialized forms of keratin. Skin cells are constantly dying, being shed and replaced by cells forming underneath. New skin cells take between two to four weeks to form and reach the surface. This skin layer helps in the protection against heat, chemicals, light, and microorganisms.

The dermis lies below the epidermis. It is mostly made up of elastic and fibrous connective tissue, and contains tiny blood and lymph vessels. This layer also contains nerve endings of sensory nerves, hair follicles, sweat glands, and oil glands. Sweat glands are controlled by the nervous system and respond to emotions as well as the body's need to lose heat. They secrete a watery fluid to help regulate the body temperature and to facilitate the excretion of wastes such as urea and salts.

Both the epidermis and the dermis contain nerve endings that can sense pain, cold, pressure and itchiness. These sensations can evoke protective reflexes or transmit pleasurable sensations such as warmth and touch. The subcutaneous layer under the dermis contains adipose tissue, which is the storage depot for fats and some blood vessels. This layer also helps in regulation of body temperature and provides cushioning to the skin.

> **Issues regarding our ability to set boundaries, be upfront, exercise authentic expression and ward off invasions, may be reflected in our skin.**

As mentioned earlier, the skin provides a variety of vital functions for our health and well-being. It is the body's first line of defence for our body against organisms and infections. An important feature of the skin, being the external boundary of the body, is that it seamlessly meets up to and communes with the mucous membranes of external body openings; at the mouth and anus of the digestive system, and at external openings to the urinary, reproductive and respiratory systems. In the skin, there exists a beautifully united orchestra of activity working to bring us safely connected to the world out there.

The Mind-Body Connection of the Skin

Our skin, particularly the skin on our face, can reflect our state of emotional and physical health. It reflects our age, diet and lifestyle choices, such as how much sleep we get, and whether we smoke or not. It reflects emotional patterns of worry, anxiety, happiness, and peacefulness. It can announce immediate emotional reactions, such as when we go red with embarrassment or anger, white with fear, or clammy with anxiety and stress. Our skin is our boundary to the outside world. Issues regarding our ability to set boundaries, be upfront, exercise authentic expression and ward off invasions, may be reflected in our skin. (Shapiro, 2006; Bourbeau, 2001)

Skin gives us sensitivity to touch. Touch is essential to life. Infants can die without it and children and adults alike cannot thrive without it. We deteriorate mentally and physically without human contact and touch. This has been documented in research done with premature babies, who will struggle to thrive when placed in incubators unless they are touched and held regularly. We touch others and we feel the touch from others through the skin. We can feel and come to know a lot about another person through their touch. Hugging and holding can be very healing, yet if touch or holding is associated with abuse we may have distorted beliefs related to touch. Our skin is very sensitive and sensuous making it a channel for our emotions. Because the skin covers the entire surface of our body, all the chakras play a role in nourishing it. However, the first three chakras, being associated with the physical body and our sense of individuality and empowerment, are especially con-

> *Our skin is very sensitive and sensuous making it a channel for our emotions.*

nected to skin issues. Shapiro (2006), states that small burns remind us of how we need to slow down. That we are trying to do too much, too quickly. Big burns are another thing. They can signify very hot emotions like anger, frustration or pain. "Big burns are a a big message that life is precious and not to burn it up." (p. 306) When we suffer a burn, we realize quickly that we cannot live comfortably without healthy skin. We lose our protective cover.

Boundaries can be an issue for many of us. It is important to honour what is comfortable for us in any given moment. It can be difficult at times to trust that we will be accepted whether or not we reach out or expose ourselves. We can learn to say no and to feel safe when we sense another invading our privacy. As trust builds, it can enlighten and release us from wariness and fear. For some of us, letting self-love and acceptance radiate into our boundary issues and invasive memories can be tough. Imagine bringing self-love and acceptance right close up to any self-doubt lurking within, and then infusing your skin with the sweetness of yourself. When allowing healthy self-respect to flow, it is easier to ward off what others may say or do that introduces self doubt.

> *Imagine letting your inner truths radiate out through your skin for all the world to see.*

Notice where you have not respected your own wishes and dreams, and allowed others to erode these and pull you out of your longing. Imagine standing in a relationship with your boundaries intact and feeling free to give and receive love without a sense of pending invasion. Perhaps that love is there for your enjoyment, being offered freely to you, and you feel free to accept it. No strings attached. Imagine that with each touch you offer and each touch you receive, love is unconditionally being transmitted.

Questions to consider

...when working with your skin.

Skin issues can arise when someone or something has crossed a boundary and gets "under your skin" or is making your "skin crawl". If you are having skin problems, you may want to consider whether you have experienced and still do experience invasions to your emotional and personal privacy.

Do you allow people to cross your boundaries against your wishes?

Are you holding back from expressing yourself freely in your life?

Can you communicate freely as if the reaction of your audience doesn't matter?

What if you were able to speak your truth and it felt safe in the face of others to allow your words to fall where they may?

Imagine that you could recognize and hear truth from others without falling apart, without your boundaries collapsing, and with a sense of holding strong allowing your skin to breath it in. Imagine letting your inner truths radiate out through your skin for all the world to see.

When your skin feels irritated, for example when you have a rash or skin infection, ask yourself who is irritating you?

What is it that you are afraid to let others see in you?

What is it you have to hold back?

Is your skin like a "mask" that you can hide behind?

Can you go out in public without makeup on?

As you consider the source of your skin problems you may want to consider relationship, and emotional factors, as well as stress, diet, chemicals or allergies.

Where Your Mind Goes Energy Flows – A Self-Healing Manual for the Mind and Body

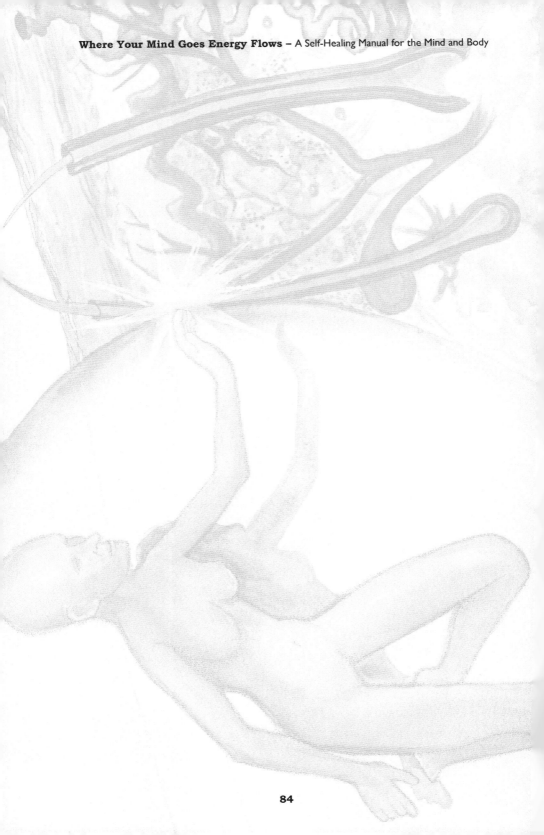

Self-Healing Meditation for the Skin System
Boundary of Reception and Protection

Bring the image of the skin into your awareness. Place your right hand on your lower belly and your left hand on your upper chest—relax and let loving healing energy flow deep into your skin and its underlying layers. Track the energy consciousness in your skin.

Let the skin's natural balancing forces of receiving and protecting come into harmony. You may want to place your hands where you are having skin problems.

Allow the skin's natural intentions to be the safe protective barrier, to regulate your temperature, to allow you to have skin sensations, to feel the loving touch of others, and to face the world confidently.

Imagine that with each touch you offer and each touch you receive, love is unconditionally being transmitted. Your skin will protect you. It is safe to hold your boundaries and you will still be loved.

Allow trust, self-love and respect to radiate out through every pore in your skin announcing to the world your loving, grand presence.

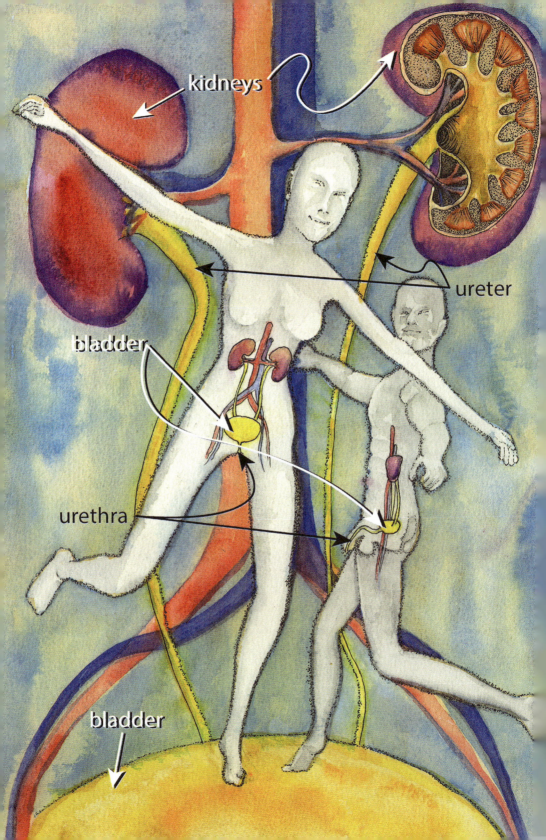

Chapter 9
The Urinary System
Elimination and Balance

The urinary system of the body is not often talked about, let alone contemplated, in our regular daily life. We often take for granted the work that the kidneys and bladder do to keep the body clean and balanced. However, we do know that when the bladder is full, it commands our attention to be relieved, often to the point that it overtakes our thoughts and ability to function normally. The kidneys are responsible for the balance of useful substances and release of the negative substances in the body.

Anatomy and Physiology of the Urinary System

As you explore the urinary system, keep in mind the concepts of release and balance that this system so gracefully carry out in concert with the rest of the body. The urinary system consists of the kidneys, the ureters, bladder and the urethra. This is where the fluids of the body are regulated and wastes can be eliminated. The three major functions of the urinary system include balancing the volume and solute concentration of the blood, removal of waste products from the blood and elimination of these waste products to the outside of the body through the bladder.

The process of balance and elimination begins as blood enters the kidneys through the renal arteries, which further divides into smaller and smaller blood vessels eventually delivering blood to filtering units called nephrons, which are exquisitely designed to regulate the concentration of essential components in the blood and filter out the wastes. These adjustments made to the blood help to regulate blood pressure and volume by controlling the amount of water and blood concentrations of sodium, potassium, chloride and other ions. The kidneys also help stabilize blood pH (acid/alkaline levels) and conserve valuable nutrients. Waste products and excess molecules are then removed from the blood, leaving it relatively free of waste products and toxins. The blood (now with the desired concentrations of many useful substances, such as glucose, water, salts and amino acids) then re-circulates back into the body. As the process continues, the urine (containing the waste products and excess water, ions and soluble components) then leaves the kidneys flowing through the ureters to the bladder. Urine is temporarily stored in the bladder until it passes through the urethra and out of the body. The creation of urine is a precise and complex process.

The Mind-Body Connection of the Urinary System

The purpose of the urinary system is to rid the body of impurities and remove substances that are no longer useful. In mind-body medicine, fluids in the body correspond to our emotions. Bladder problems are often said to be related to being angry or perhaps better said, "being pissed-off" about something.

> *Could the urinary system be connected to negative emotions?*

Long-standing resentments can develop when you fear that reprisals will occur if you release negative feelings. You may have childhood experiences of disapproval for expressing negative feelings such crying or whining. It may be that you never learned how to express your negative thoughts and feelings without parental disapproval.

Could problems with the urinary system be connected to a difficulty in one's ability to release negative emotions? Urinary infections often occur during the stress of relationship trauma, when negativity runs high and when conflicts arise that are difficult to express. We may feel during these times that we are losing our individuality and are feeling pressure to conform. The kidneys are also considered the "seat of fear" in Chinese medicine. They are closely connected to the adrenal glands which sit right on top of the kidneys. Adrenal glands release adrenalin in the face of fear, stress, anger, panic or excitement. Dr. Shapiro (2006) states that the kidneys are affected by unexpressed fear and grief. According to Choa Kok Sui (1992) in his writings about advanced pranic healing he states that malfunctions in the first, second and third chakras can lead to urinary problems. The whole system is energized by the second chakra. The third chakra influences the kidneys, and the first chakra nourishes the bladder. He goes on to say that "In certain cases, long-standing deep resentment in the form of congested red pranic energy from the solar plexus or third chakra goes down to the kidneys, thereby causing them to malfunction. This is why, in some instances, long-standing negative emotions may severely damage the kidneys." (p. 201)

Difficulties in the urinary system may be connected to the inability to release the negativity in our lives. Recognizing and releasing negative emotions may support the urinary system to relax and carry out its purpose of removing impurities and supporting balance within the body. The natural ebb and flow of positive and negative emotions is an ongoing life experience.

Questions to consider

...when working with your urinary system.

Do you have a tendency to keep your feelings bottled-up?

Is it difficult to speak up clearly and release negative emotions?

What childhood traumas have eroded your trust and have caused you to fear letting go of negativity?

What emotions do you feel hostage to that block you in life?

Is fear or anxiety a predominant issue in your life?

> Fears about disapproval and rejection may, cause one to hold on to, rather than communicate negative thoughts and feelings.

Do you often feel panicky, worried or anxious?

In your childhood was it difficult to express negative thoughts and feelings without parental disapproval?

Fears about disapproval and rejection may, cause one to hold on to, rather than communicate negative thoughts and feelings.

Each person in a relationship comes to the table with their own personal family culture of expressing or withholding negative emotions. It would be helpful to identify what your family customs are and how they have helped or harmed the release of emotions in your life. It takes courage and practice to share negative thoughts and feelings with an intimate partner, friend, co-worker or family member and still hold love and acceptance for each other. Freely expressing positive and negative emotions may support the urinary system's function of balance and elimination.

Self-Healing Meditation for
the Urinary System
Elimination and Balance

Bring the image of the urinary system to your awareness. Place your right hand on your lower belly to connect to your bladder, and your left hand on the your upper belly to connect to the kidneys. Let energy flow from your hands with tenderness throughout this system.

As you explore the urinary system, keep in mind the release and balance that this system so gracefully carries out to support the body.

Notice if you are holding on to any long-standing fear, resentment or anger. Allow trust and self-love to flow and nourish the urinary system. You can release negative emotions and long-standing resentments gently over time as trust is built up.

Let energy flow into the bladder, the kidneys and adrenal glands to dissolve any negativity happening. Allow the natural ebb and flow of positive and negative emotions to be restored.

Simply trust in the purity of the urinary system in its ability to remove impurities and balance the body fluids and chemicals with harmony and flow.

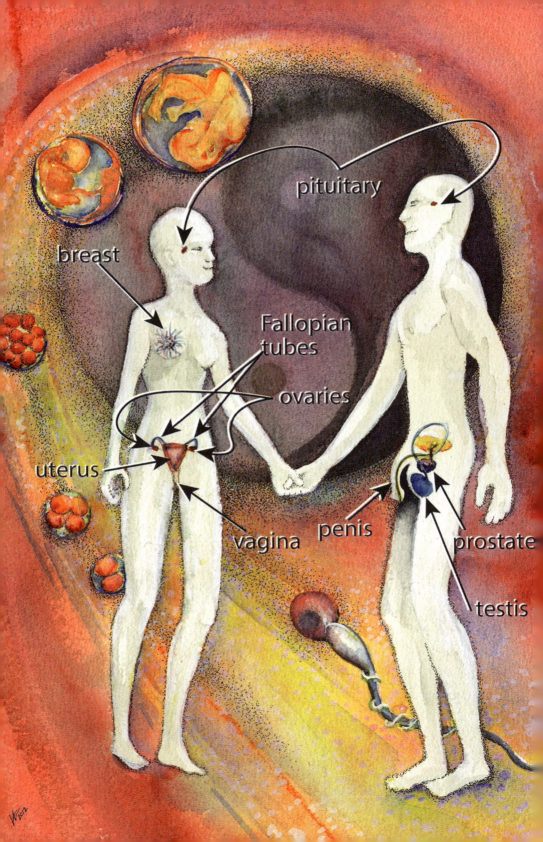

Chapter 10
The Reproductive System
Creativity and Sexuality

Imagine that, regardless of how we identify as male, female or something entirely different, we all have both feminine and masculine characteristics. Each of us is made up of a unique blend of masculine and feminine forces which when unrestricted, support a balanced creative consciousness through which to live our lives. Let's explore this fascinating body system in more detail.

Anatomy and Physiology of the Reproductive System

The male and female sexual organs along with the pituitary gland, produce the hormones necessary for the proper development, maintenance, and functioning of the organs of reproduction, and other organs and tissues in the body. The ovaries and testes develop during puberty and become active under the influence of the pituitary gland, resulting in the production of sex hormones; testosterone in males and estrogen and progesterone in females. In both the male and female, these hormones are directly involved in the development of the sexual characteristics and processes of the body.

Reproduction is the process of producing a child. From a purely scientific point of view, reproduction is for the survival of the species, passing on hereditary traits from one generation to the next. The male and female reproductive systems contribute to the events leading to fertilization and conception. The reproductive organs are critical to the creation of the next generation. Together, the sperm from the father and the ovum from the mother form the genetic matrix for the new being to express itself through. The mother then assumes responsibility for the developing the baby. Together the mother and father take on the role of parenting. It seems very straightforward when you look at it this way. As we know, there are many other factors involved in this process, not the least of which are the pyscho-emotional ones.

The Female Reproductive System

In the female body, the reproductive organs include the breasts, uterus, fallopian tubes, ovaries, vagina and vulva. The ovaries produce eggs which contain genetic material that gives the child some of their mother's characteristics. The eggs then travel through the fallopian tubes to the uterus for fertilization. The menstrual cycle is hormonally regulated by a very sophisticated feedback system for the monthly cyclical production of eggs. When an egg is fertilized by sperm, another feedback system comes into play. The hormones that are released support the growth of the fetus and support the person's body during pregnancy and for breastfeeding.

The uterus is pear-shaped and has muscular walls and a thick lining of tissue. It is here that the fetus begins to grow. The muscles of the uterus protect the fetus and are able to expand to accommodate its increasing size. At the baby's time of birth, under the influence of an amazing process of hormonal direction, the uterine muscles contract and push the baby out into the world. The breasts can play the very important role of producing milk and providing a vessel for feeding the infant. However, the breasts also play a very sensual role in sexual expression and sexual identity.

Later in life during menopause, there is a natural change and reduction in the secretion of hormones. This presents females with a whole new, and sometimes challenging, host of symptoms, including the cessation of the menstrual cycle and the ability to conceive.

Male Reproductive System

A male's reproductive organs include the testes, accessory ducts, accessory glands, and penis. Most of the male reproductive organs are external including the testes and penis. The accessory glands and ducts are internal. Sperm and testosterone are produced in the testicles which sit outside of the body in the scrotal sac. Sperm contain chromosomes that carry the genetic blueprint determining the paternally inherited characteristics and the sex of the child. Testosterone is the hormone that supports the masculine influence on the body. The penis is part of the male reproductive system as well as the urinary system. When sexually aroused, the penis becomes erect as the erectile tissue fills with blood. When the penis is erect the male is ready for sexual intercourse and able to eject sperm via a fluid called seminal fluid. This fluid is produced by three glands, one of which is the prostate gland. The prostate gland is closely connected to the urinary system, and when enlarged, can affect the flow of urine through the penis. Erectile dysfunctions are closely linked to emotional as well as physical issues. Here we find a very curious example of the mind-body connection. Most erectile dysfunction treatment plans include addressing psychological issues.

The Pituitary Gland

The pituitary gland is found at the base of the brain and is one centimetre in diametre. The reproductive system is dependent on it as it secretes hormones that stimulate the onset of puberty and the ongoing functions of the male and female reproductive organs, including pregnancy. These hormones, in their proper balance and timing, support the healthy functioning and purpose of human reproduction and the expression of our sexuality. The pituitary gland also secretes other hormones that affect other parts of the human body discussed in the chapter on the endocrine system.

The Mind-Body Connection of the Reproductive System

As mentioned, the reproductive system is about creation and the expression of our sexuality. As humans, we naturally have a deep drive to produce and offer our creations to humanity passing them down through the generations. Through the process of conception, fetal development and child rearing, we pass on hereditary traits, belief

> *Can a healthy reproductive system support us in our continuous desire to create?*

systems, physical traits, habits, customs and thought forms from one generation to the next. The health of the male and female reproductive systems are obviously integral to the creation of a healthy baby. Can a healthy reproductive system support us in our continuous desire to create with passion and excitement, be it a work of art, a relationship or a gourmet meal, let alone a baby? Can a lack of self-love or negative beliefs about our sexuality affect the health of our reproductive system?

The reproductive system resides mostly within the energy consciousness of the second chakra. The second chakra embodies the consciousness of self-love and the feelings we have about ourselves as a woman, a man, or a combination of both. Carolyn Myss (1997) describes the energy anatomy of the second chakra as it relates to emotional issues around money, sex, power and control. Shapiro (2006) discusses the emotional underpinnings of our sexuality as they relate to self-worth, self-like or dislike.

Yin and yang, the Chinese reference to the nature of the feminine (yin) and masculine (yang), is inherent in every human being regardless of their gender.

She explains that our feelings about ourselves as a sexual being are influenced by the quality of our first relationships, such as with our parents. There is a strong connection between how we love and accept ourselves and how we treat others. Relationships are certainly affected by our sense of ourselves as sexual, creative and passionate beings. Furthermore, we deal with the strong stereotypes ingrained in our society (that vary from culture to culture) about what it means to be a man or a woman. Generational sexual stereotypes, negative belief systems about sex and passion can influence our sexual health.

Many of us have never even entertained the idea that we all possess a unique personal blend of both yin and yang.

For the creative flow to unfold fully, it requires a combination of both masculine and feminine qualities of expression. Yin and yang, the Chinese reference to the nature of the feminine (yin) and masculine (yang), is inherent in every human being regardless of their gender. Many of us have never even entertained the idea that we all possess a unique personal blend of both yin and yang. The feminine and masculine principles qualify power in different ways. The yang or masculine principle expresses itself in an outward, goal-directed and straight-forward path to defeat adversity. In contrast, the yin or feminine principle expresses itself in an inward journey to embrace and be with the adversity, to understand it and allow solutions to unfold. The feminine journey seeks a more circular and relational approach to self-discovery, assertiveness and power. Together, the feminine and the masculine principles support and facilitate power and creativity.

> *Together, the feminine and the masculine principles support and facilitate power and creativity.*

If one takes a closer look at our activities and expressions each day, in them lies the yin and yang qualities working in tandem. Some activities may require more of a traditionally feminine emphasis, such as perhaps dancing, and other activities may require more of a traditionally masculine approach, such as driving a car, but neither activity is completely exclusive to one or the other. Living our life supported by the wisdom of feminine and masculine principles can help us to grow into a place of inner authority with grace, strength, creativity and passion.

Questions to consider

...when working with your reproductive system.

An inability to harness both energies when required often leads to problems and lifelong difficulties.

For example, in certain relationships do you tend to be more focused on the outcome and the future and always seek or force direct action?

Do you let the feminine principle express itself and embrace the adversities that arise, allowing yourself to let solutions unfold?

Do you avoid taking decisive goal-directed actions when required?

Do you trust a more feminine or masculine approach to life?

How do you approach your career, parenting, and even your leisure time?

Do you trust in your sexuality?

Can you trust in your creative flow?

Do you know and trust in what you are passionate about?

Can you love, accept and enjoy your sexual orientation?

What childhood traumas have deteriorated your ability to accept yourself and create with freedom?

Is there some history of sexual abuse in your life or in your family tree?

Have others respected your sexual boundaries?

Was it customary in your family to ignore sexual improprieties and abuse that occurred in the family?

Was it "bad" to point out any suspected or actual known incidences of sexual abuse in your family?

Was this considered disrespectful to the family?

Sexual abuse can dampen one's ability to be passionate or creative in life to say the least. Sexual repression or abuse can lead to severe self-disrespect, self-mistrust and self-hatred. Overtime, without any healing, sexual abuse can cause a variety of problems, such as submissiveness or aggressive behaviour, repeated relationship difficulties, depression and physical disorders of the reproductive system.

In the field of energy medicine, feminine energy is said to be sourced from the left side of the body and masculine energy from the right side. This is an interesting thought as we think about how to balance our feminine and masculine energies.

Which side of your body do you tend to ignore?

Which side of your body is weaker, gets injured more often or is less developed?

Do you tend to value one sex over the other?

As full bodied humans in our quest for unity on this earth, we are called to understand both forces, to know and be able to exercise both the feminine and the masculine dynamics of power and influence within ourselves, in a respectful and balanced fashion. Living in one's truth with a personal balance of yin and yang is the essence of self-power and divine self-realization. Perhaps as each of us attempts to understand both our feminine and masculine selves, we can begin to help heal the separation of the genders and other expressions of duality that exist so deeply in our world today.

Where Your Mind Goes Energy Flows – A Self-Healing Manual for the Mind and Body

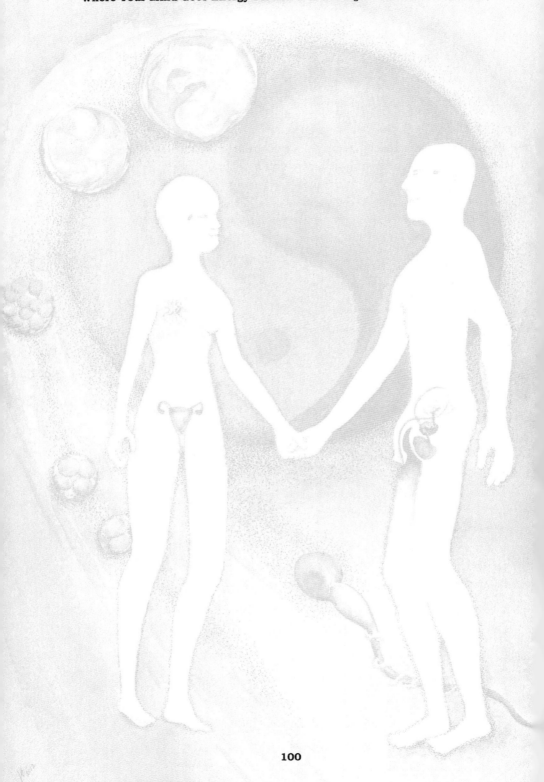

Self-Healing Meditation for the Reproductive System
Creativity and Sexuality

Bring the image of the reproductive system into your awareness. Place your right hand on your lower belly to connect to your reproductive organs, and your left hand on your upper chest or lightly holding the bridge of your nose to connect with the pituitary gland in the brain. Let loving energy flow through your hands to this system.

What is it you long to create?

Notice any feelings you have about your sexuality—what it means to be a woman, a man or the gender you identify with. Hold these feelings with understanding and tenderness.

Simply trust in the purity of the reproductive system and in its ability to bring the hormonal cycles into rhythm.

Allow your reproductive system to relax into a state of self-love with its creative abilities and natural sexuality.

Allow the feminine and masculine principles to flow through you, strengthening your authentic inner authority with grace, creativity and passion. Let the reproductive system's creative forces come into harmony and balance.

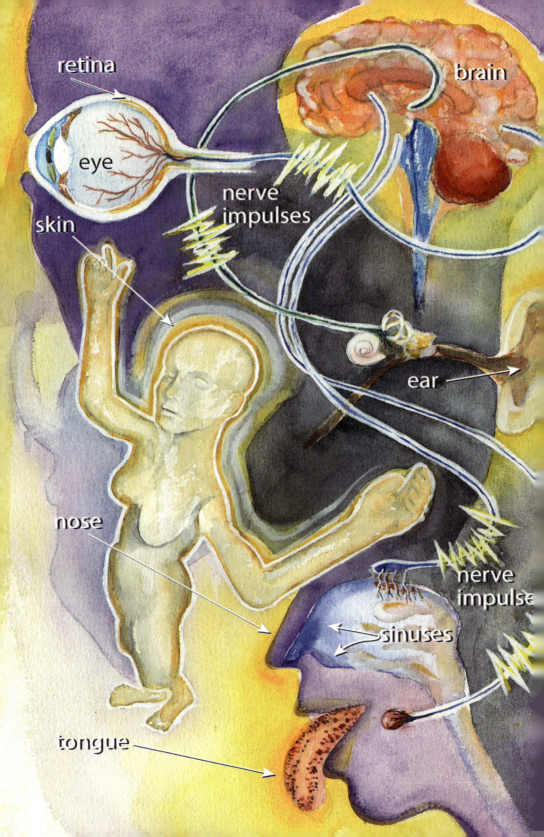

Chapter 11
The Sensory System
Perceiving and Discerning

The senses of hearing, smell, sight and taste and our ability to speak and express ourselves, brings us into intimate connection and communication with the world around us. Our senses provide us with a tool to penetrate into the nature of reality. We can then respond with more accuracy to our environment including the people with whom we connect.

Anatomy and Physiology of the Sensory System

Sense of Hearing—The Ears

The ears are exquisitely designed to collect, direct and detect minute vibrations in the air. These vibrations are directed through the outer ear and then transformed in the middle and inner ear into electrical impulses that travel to the brain. This system gives us the ability to hear sounds and to interpret them through the brain. The ears also play a role in the sense of balance. As you know, every time you stand or sit up, you must balance yourself. Even when you walk, jump, or move around you are always balancing yourself. The inner ear contains small circular tubes filled with fluid to accomplish this task. How ingenious!

Sense of Smell—The Nose

The nose has receptors that perceive chemical stimuli that produce olfactory sensations (the sense of smell). It has a remarkable built-in scent recognition, processing and memory recording system. Smell is probably one of the most primitive senses, and it is also the one most directly connected to the subconscious layers of the psyche and of memory. It is the one sense that triggers memories the most. A simple scent is enough to relive a scene from the past and to feel all the emotions associated with it. Along with the job of smelling, the nose also does a wonderful job of receiving the air we breathe. The bony and cartilaginous structure of the nasal passages is designed for easy flow of air into the rest of the air passages. When the nasal passages are healthy the sense of smell works well.

Sense of Taste—The Tongue

The tongue is made of muscle tissue and its surface has receptors that perceive chemical stimuli that produce tasting sensations. The tongue has numerous taste buds allowing us to discern a myriad of tastes. Often, in order to taste something we also have to smell it. These two senses work together in many cases. In fact, the olfactory receptors can detect substances much smaller than the taste buds can, and this gives us a vast range of tasting possibilities.

Sense of Sight—The Eyes

The eyes give us the precious sense of sight. Like the other sensory organs, they miraculously transform sensory stimuli into nerve signals that travel to the brain allowing us to understand what we see. The eyes sit in the protective eye sockets of the skull and are moved by six delicate muscles. The eyes receive light rays that reflect off objects in our line of vision. These rays of light are transmitted onto the retina at the back of the eye. The retina is a delicate layer of tissue and is made up of millions of rod and cone cells. These retinal cells convert the images received into nerve signals, which travel to the brain for inter-

> *We perceive the world around us through a cone of perception which is influenced by our upbringing, unresolved conflicts, everyday experiences as well as our community, family customs and ancestral heritage.*

pretation. The brain receives and processes visual information on a continual basis, tracking the changing images. The eyes also contain many tiny tear-secreting and mucus-forming glands that protect the eyes from damage due to dryness.

Speaking—The Larynx or Voice Box

The larynx is a structure in the neck that governs our voice. No two voices are the same, just as no two faces are the same. The production of sound is dependent on the flow of air through the voice box.

The Mind-Body Connection of the Sensory System

It can be difficult to actively listen to others or to ourselves when we are distracted by issues and judgments. From a psycho-emotional perspective, difficulties in hearing may be related to the inability to cope with family conflict (in present circumstances or in your past). It may also be that you feel you have never been heard by others or are afraid of hearing your own voice. We all have an inherent need to be heard, acknowledged and recognized; to feel whole, worthy and loved. (Hay, 1998; Shapiro, 2006; Myss, 1997)

The way we use our voice conveys a great deal about our personality. It offers us a beautiful means of expression for sharing who we are with the world. Expression depends largely on tone and intent more than on the words we choose. It is often said that the tone in our voice speaks much louder than our words. Children are very sensitive to tone versus words, particularly before they have learned to speak. (Shapiro, 2006; Myss, 1997)

To speak truthfully, and to be open to hearing truth, requires a clear and uninterrupted flow of information from the outside world, as well as from our own of thoughts and feelings. We perceive the world around us through a filter we can call a "cone of perception". Our perceptions are influenced by our upbringing, unresolved conflicts, everyday experiences, our community, family customs and ancestral heritage. It is through this cone of perception that we understand and deal with life.

The nose senses beautiful scents and repugnant doors alike. Its remarkable built-in scent recognition, processing and memory recording system allows us to be transported back into memories with one whiff. Scents are often associated with emotions. We even use our nose to sense what is going on, like when we sense something is wrong and we "smell a rat." It can also be a tool that we use to poke our way into other people's business—like when we are being "nosey." (Shapiro, 2006) In general, the area around the ears, nose, mouth and throat are governed by the fifth chakra. Carolyn Myss (1997) refers to fifth chakra issues as being about choice and strength of will; personal expression and following one's dream. Barbara Brennan (1993) explains that speaking one's truth, and the ability to give and receive, is related to a healthy energy flow of the fifth chakra.

Our eyes are the windows to our soul—to our inner being. Just like we can see and know the feelings of others through their eyes, they can also see and know our feelings. The eyes are nourished by the energy of the sixth chakra. The sixth chakra governs the ability to have vision and foresight. (Myss, 1997) Distorted energy in this chakra may be seen in those who lack self-awareness or a sense of spiritual connectedness. This can result in a fear of the inner self and lead to distorted images of reality. Brennan (1993) explains further that the sixth chakra governs the left eye and the seventh chakra governs the right eye. Both these energy centres feed our intellectual abilities, our ability to evaluate ourselves, to learn from experience and allow us to be open to the ideas of others. Clear sight is dependent on a healthy brain as this is where images are interpreted. Difficulties with sight may be a reflection of childhood emotional trauma, leading to fears and withdrawal from the outside world. Eye problems may suggest an inability to accept what you see happening in your life. (Shapiro, 2006; Hay, 1998) Sight is more than just seeing. The sense of sight comes with feelings, perceptions, and a sense of knowing. Many times we see and interpret events from our limited belief systems about life. We may be unable to understand the perceptions of others because we "see" things differently.

Questions to consider

...when working with your sensory system.

What are you refusing to hear?

Are you turning a deaf ear to your own needs?

Do you always put others first, even denying your own needs?

Are you out of balance in your life?

A healthy sense of hearing may involve listening to our own inner voice about our own needs and feelings.

Are you able to speak up for yourself?

What does the quality of your voice say about you?

Do you have difficulty communicating from your authentic sense of self?

Can you identify your listening patterns?

How are you listening or speaking from a learned pattern in your family?

What critical voices do you hear inside your mind that come from your parents or other authority figures?

Do you sometimes hear yourself speaking with automatic critical comments to yourself or others?

Are you turning a blind eye to your own needs?

Can your tears flow easily?

Do you use your glasses as a shield? Do you feel defenceless or exposed when you take them off?

Can you see the divine in yourself; in others?

What are you seeing or perceiving that is upsetting?

What truths do you refuse to see in your life, in your family or ancestral heritage?

What needs to be brought out into the light of the day?

Self-Healing Meditation for the Sensory System
Perceiving and Discerning

Bring the images of the sensory system to your awareness. Place your hands on each side of your head, above or in front of your ears. Allow energy to flow from your hands to the sensory organs and to sensory centres in the brain.

Sense how the energy consciousness is flowing. Notice if the flow gets blocked.

Allow warmth, trust and love to flow into the sensory system to balance and restore health to your eyes, nose, mouth, tongue, voice box and ears, including connections to the sensory centres within the brain.

Allow the sensory system to take in and accurately sense various stimuli. Notice any sounds, tastes, images or words that come to you.

Your sensory organs are masters at gently and accurately receiving, perceiving and interpreting information from your surroundings.

Support the sensory system's ability to communicate accurate messages to the brain. Take a deep breath and relax into your senses.

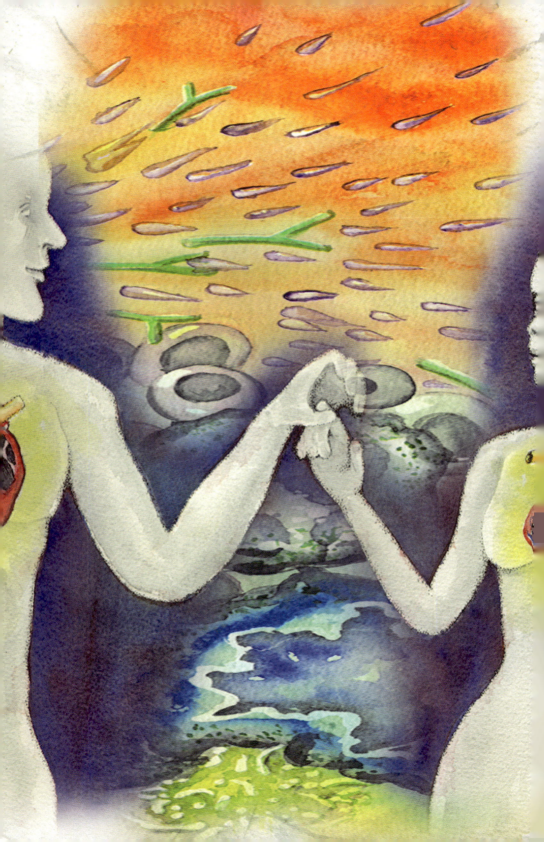

Chapter 12
The Whole Body

This meditation is a simple and effective way to generally support your mind-body health and augment the self-healing meditations in the previous chapter exercises.

Your body and mind is always seeking homeostasis, balance and health. Our cells are very receptive and perceptive to the environment around us, as well as to our state of inner being.

In this exercise, you are rebooting your cells into a healthy working order. You are informing and directing the energy particles, at the quantum level, on how to behave.

Set your intention for this self-healing.

What do you long for?

What do want for this healing?

Self-Healing Meditation for the Whole Body

Lie or sit quietly and place your left hand on your heart and your right hand on your lower belly. Relax and breathe. Bring awareness to your body starting at your feet moving up to your head. Notice any physical sensations and breathe with them. As the healing progresses, feel free to place your hands anywhere on the body that you feel needs healing.

Let any thoughts and emotions (the stuff of life) come up and float up off of your body. Simply observe them and let them flow past. If thoughts cycle back—acknowledge them and then invite them to float on by. You may want to imagine that you are like a riverbed, and the stuff of life is in the river water, that flows over you.

Access your core light within—the part of you that knows no age—that feels the same whether you are 3, or 30, or 60, or 90! This "light" often feels excited, relaxed, positive and full of possibilities.

Take some time to bring your awareness to any problem you might be having. It may be an emotional issue, relationship issue, physical symptom or spiritual question. With your imagination, direct loving energy into the problem area. Breathe. Relax and observe what comes up in your mind and body. Trust that simply observing and loving yourself in the moment will begin the healing process. Bless yourself, and make a statement for the healing you desire.

To close, imagine your personal, sweet core light expanding and filling your body, penetrating every cell. Then let your light expand out around you, into the room, house, neighbourhood, city, country and over all of the earth. Let it flow as far as it feels comfortable.

The healing energy will continue to work even after you are finished. You can fall asleep or go about your day.

Your ability to focus and sink into your innate healing powers will build over time. Be patient with yourself. Above all, enjoy yourself.

You are the healer and the healed.

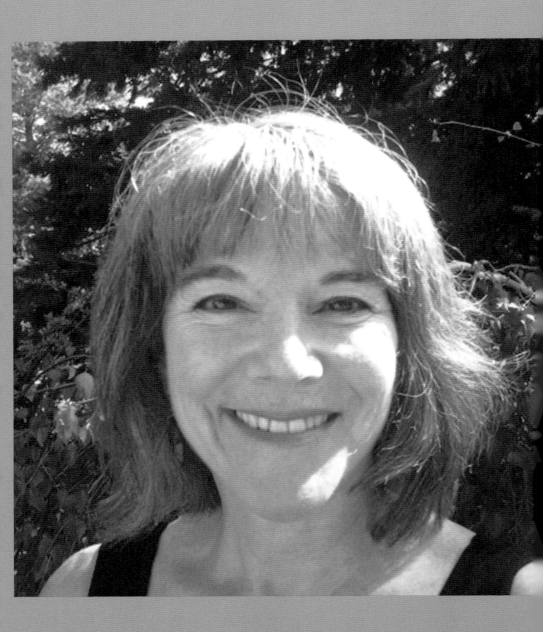

Conclusion

I have always been completely enamoured by the body's ability to heal. It is a beautiful healing machine. It is always seeking, homeostasis and whole health. I encourage you to practice supporting your body to heal with these body system meditations. It will become easier each time you try them. I encourage you to be patient with yourself. It takes time for some of us to learn to focus loving energy into the physical body. I encourage you to be creative with this work. You may want to draw your own versions of the mind-body systems. You may want to assign certain colours or feelings to each mediation or try certain songs or sounds to help heal your mind and body systems. Do not hold yourself back. Humanity is continually evolving and we are all learning new ways to heal ourselves. Energy healing is becoming mainstream. Meditation is becoming mainstream.

I want to close with a personal account of an experience I had in my fourth year at the Barbara Brennan School of Healing. During this experience, it felt as though everything was made of energy, even solid inanimate objects. This sea of energy was fluid and dynamic, albeit less so in dense forms, but nonetheless in flux. I was a part of the sea of energy and the unifying feeling, I would say, was all-knowing LOVE.

Here is my journal entry of May, 2002.

"I had an unbelievable experience that materialized out of nowhere in my supervision session with Kate last week. I was struggling with feeling invaded by negative energy from family, and depleted from "doing" so much in my life for others—having so much on my plate—not caring for myself enough. We were talking about presencing from my core and then Kate asked me something that triggered my "dropping" into this feeling. She asked me "What if you never do another healing?" This stopped me in my tracks and I dropped into a place. In this place, I truly had an exquisite attentiveness to the now…with no thoughts of attachment to anything. I knew I was in my bedroom but then I didn't really know that this was my bedroom. I was enamoured with the wooden bedposts on my bed and the wooden furniture around me, and yet I couldn't tell them apart from each other or from the walls or the sheets. I thought about people. I felt as though everyone and everything was connected and all was ONE, including the bedposts. Each object I looked at was beautiful and was a part of my life and not part of my life. I was spirit and I was flesh. I was not separate from other people or other beings and in some way I could feel I was. My cells were glowing and the feeling of POTENTIAL was everywhere—even in the inanimate objects around me! Things came in and out of my perception – with no attachments at all. I don't think I would have understood the word attachment at this point in time. Time meant nothing at all. I could walk—I tried this. I could turn my head from side to side but this happened VERY slowly. I felt bliss I guess, but it didn't matter that it was bliss. This state of being lasted for about 15 to 20 minutes then the wave of it slowly lessened.

The words that I want to identify with this experience are, ENDURING and PERVASIVE LOVE, UNTETHERED POTENTIAL, UNITY, TIMELESSNESS, ONENESS, MOMENT TO MOMENT JOURNEYING. In this place, no one or no thing needs healing."

This experience gave me a glimpse into the meaning of universal love: love without conditions, love that is eternal, steady, pervasive and completely reliable. It felt as though love was the backdrop from which all 'life' is launched. I remember that in the afternoon, right after this experience, I put my jacket on, gathered my car keys and purse and went to pick up my kids at school with such a wide-open heart full of love. I could not wait to see them.

We are all
made of,
and
come from,
love.

Our cells
thrive
in an
atmosphere
of
love.

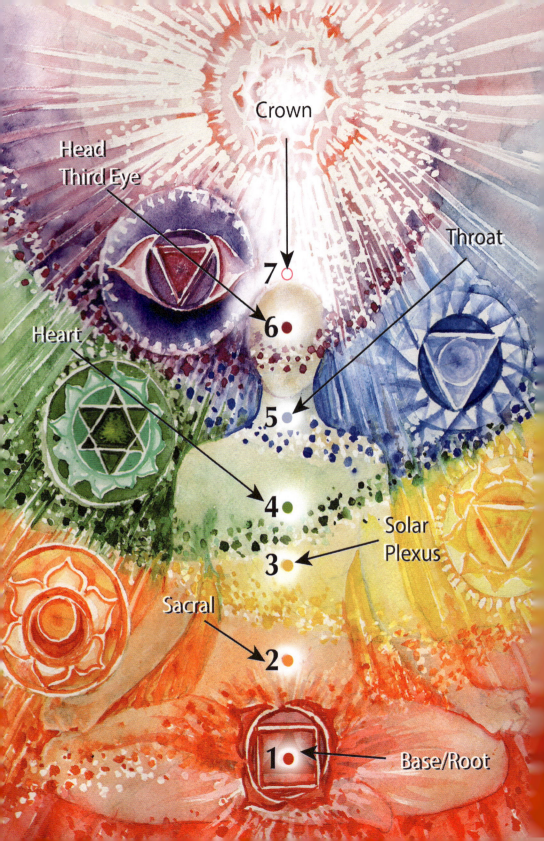

Appendix
Chakras

The location of the seven major chakras are illustrated in this image along with the colours associated with each of their vibrations.

Chakras exchange energy with the universal energy field to nourish your personal energy field within and around the body. They are cone-shaped vortices that funnel energy consciousness into the front and the back of the body. In this frontal image you can see where they are located. The more healthy energy we let flow, the healthier we are. A lack of energy flowing can lead to disease and distorts our experience of life.

"Since this energy is always associated with a form of consciousness, we experience the energy we exchange in terms of seeing, hearing, feeling, sensing, intuiting or direct knowing," (Brennan, 1988, p.45)

1. Base/Foot
2. Sacral
3. Solar Plexus
4. Heart
5. Throat
6. Head/Third Eye
7. Crown

References

Amen, D. G. (1998). *Change your brain change your life. The breakthrough program for conquering anxiety, depression, obsessiveness, anger, and impulsiveness.* New York: Three Rivers Press.

Bourbeau, L. (2001). *Your body is telling you: Love yourself. The most complete book on metaphysical causes of illness and disease.* Saint-Jerome, QC: Les Editions E.T.C. Inc.

Brennan, B. (1988). *Hands of Light.* New York: Bantam Books.

Brennan, B. (1993). *Light Emerging. The Journey of Personal Healing.* New York: Bantam Books.

Brennan, B. (2017). *Core light healing. My personal journey and advanced healing concepts for creating the life you long to live.* United States of America: Hay House.

Dale, C. (2009). *The subtle body. An encyclopedia of your energetic anatomy.* Boulder, CO: Sounds True Inc.

Doidge, N. (2007). *The brain that changes itself. Stories of personal triumph from the frontiers of brain science.* Australia: Penguin Books.

Eden, D. (1998). *Energy medicine.* New York: Penguin Putnam Inc.

Hay, L. L. (1998). *Heal your body A-Z. Mental causes for physical illness and the way to overcome them.* Carlsbad, CA: Hay House Inc.

HeartMath Institute. (April 22, 2013). *The heart's intuitive intelligence: A path to personal, social and global coherence.* Video file. retrieved from http://www.heartmath.org.

Kenyon, T. (April 18, 2005). *Ecstasy and the heart.* (Hathor Channeling). Retrieved from http://tomkenyon.com/ecstasy-and-the-heart.

References

Maté, G. (2004). *When the body says no.* Toronto: Random House of Canada Ltd.

Myss, C. (1997). *Why don't people heal and how they can.* New York: Crown Publishing Company.

Northrup, C. (2003). *The wisdom of menopause.* New York: Bantam Books.

Pearsall, P. (1998). *The heart's code.* New York: Broadway Books.

Shapiro, D. (2006). *Your body speaks your mind. Decoding the emotional, psychological, and spiritual messages that underlie illness.* Boulder, CO: Sounds True, Inc.

Sui, C.K. (1992). *Advanced Pranic Healing Institute for Inner Studies Inc.* Manila, Philippines.

Weil, A. (1998). *Natural health, natural medicine. A comprehensive manual for wellness and self care.* Boston: Houghton Mifflin Company.

West, B. (April 16, 2014). *Proof the human body is a projection of consciousness.* Retrieved from http://www.wakingtimes.com/2014/04/16/proof-human-body-projection-consciousness/

Wolf, S. (Producer), Becker, G. (Director). (2009). *The living matrix. The science of healing.* (DVD). United States.

Zukav, G., & Francis, L. (2001). *The heart of the soul. Emotional awareness.* New York: Simon & Schuster Source.

Self-Healing Meditation Cards 12-Piece Set

available at

The Turning Point – Michèle Bourgeois B.Sc.N., M.Ed.

www.turningpointhealing.com

This is a twelve card set of 4" X 6" cards on high gloss heavy stock with colour custom art on the front along with information and a guided meditation for that respective body system on the back. These sets are an excellent tool to assist in restoring physical, mental and spiritual balance. Great for individuals seeking their own healing and health care practitioners, such as energy healers, nurses, doctors, physical therapists and massage therapists.

Each card allows one to consider the anatomy and physiology of the physical body and psycho-spiritual meaning of each body system in a holistic way. Holding onto healthful energy consciousness, specific to each body system, can help with the connection to the healing vibrations that you or your client requires.

Client Comments

"These meditations are absolutely beautiful, both conceptually, and in every detail. The artwork is so creative, and lovely to behold. There is a real synergy between the descriptions and meditations of the various systems, and the art. The illustrations are also a great visualization aid. I am keeping "The Heart & Circulation (Love & Connection)" close at hand! I had not thought of the heart as it having its own nervous system, or of the signals it sends being influenced by its owner's emotions before." (Whitehorse, Yukon 2017)

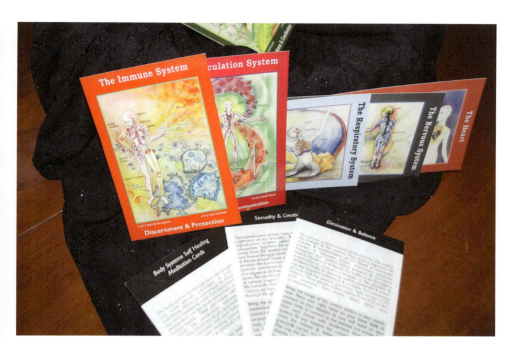

ISBN: 978-1-7751844-3-0

"I have used the Self-Healing meditation cards and found them very helpful in helping me to focus on and appreciate each system, I asked my nephew who is a firefighter/paramedic to have a look, he really liked the simple clear explanations of the body systems. Also asked my reflexologist, she really liked them and wondered if we could use the cards for me to reflect on each body system as she's working on them." (Victoria, BC 2017)

"What a great way to inform and have us all honour all the systems that give us the gift of life." (Saskatoon, SK 2017)

Made in the USA
Columbia, SC
28 January 2018